My Race Against Death

I AM NOT MY DISEASE

LESSONS LEARNED FROM MY HEALTH STRUGGLES

Shoba Rao

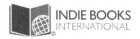

INDIE BOOKS
INTERNATIONAL

ISBN-13: 978-1-957651-25-5

Library of Congress Control Number: 2022923987

Designed by *the*BookDesigners
Illustrations by Suresh Sankralingam

INDIE BOOKS INTERNATIONAL®, INC.
2511 WOODLANDS WAY
OCEANSIDE, CA 92054
www.indiebooksintl.com

Dedication

When she was born, she was a bundle of joy,
With chubby cheeks and bright black eyes;
She instantly became my favorite toy,
And I always protected her from imaginary foes;

To the school she would scamper,
And did her math without a whimper;
That, made me feel shy, as I was much older,
And was still getting used to the books and binder;

She would listen to the radio,
And understand the plays on the audio;
She would explain the plot with glee,
All this, when she was just a few months over three!

She once jumped off a wall,
And her forehead was cracked and torn;
She felt so proud about the fall,
That she got stitched without a single moan!

It felt great to have a little sister,
Whom you could boss over like a Mister;
She has been my friend, my buddy,
For all these wonderful years steady;

She has gotten over a lot of obstacles,
And made it to where she really deserves;
May God bless my dear little sister,
Whom I love and shall cherish forever!

-Hema Rao

Contents

Preface

Every time cancer tried to grab me with its claws, I recognized anew the importance of being one step ahead in the game and fighting the right battles while running my race for life. I realized that being my own advocate is essential. After many friends approached me for advice when one of their loved ones or friends were stricken with cancer, I decided it would be good to share my story with all the lessons I learned in my journey.

Being a kidney transplant recipient for twenty-four years taught me the importance of organ donation and that, along with surviving cancer has molded me into the person I am today. In this book, I discuss my experiences and how they have changed me with the hope that the lessons from my journey will help others face the brutal world of diseases.

As an avid book reader, I recognized there weren't many stories out there like mine. Even my doctors consider my case history to be unique. I suppose few with my history have survived to tell it, which is one of the main reasons for sharing my story. This book is for all patients who would hopefully gain some insight on how to tackle a disease like cancer both physically and emotionally. I have also provided some simple nutritious recipes using superfoods.

I want to thank all my family and friends who have been with me every step of my journey, with special thanks to my mother who gave me a second chance at life by donating her organ and to my husband who remains my pillar of support to this day.

1 Childhood

Every Fighter Needs Someone In Their Corner

I WOKE UP in the middle of night shouting for my mother, "I want Amma." Even at thirty, when I was in pain, the heart called for mother. Suresh, my husband, consoled me and helped me through the pain.

My mother is just 4'10". But in my eyes, she towered tall as someone who looked after and protected me, but also as someone who did not shy away from disciplining me.

SOMEONE WAS ALWAYS IN MY CORNER

Fighting for your life is like combat. In combat sports, such as boxing and wrestling, a corner man is a person whose job is to assist the combatant between rounds. I was lucky to have two in my corner: my mother and my husband.

For every single occurrence of cancer and during all my treatments, my mother was always beside me along with my husband. She braved traveling alone with the minimal English that she knew, all the way from India, with a stopover at a busy airport on the way. During chemo, the only food that was soothing for me was food cooked by my mother.

Between my parents, she was the bad cop and dad usually played the good cop. Despite playing the bad cop it was very evident that she loved her children tremendously and always took extra care to feed us well and to protect us.

My mother was quite unaware of worldly affairs. Yet, her love for her child drove her to agree to be my donor, the day she learned of my kidney failure. The same mother who I was afraid of, who I thought was ignorant was ready to do anything to save her child.

After marriage, my husband Suresh, the love of my life, was there with me every step of the way, through thick and thin, never missing a doctor's appointment. In our twenty-two years of married life, we have had lots of memorable, gratifying, fun moments and he has made my living worthwhile despite the health hurdles. The most memorable moment in my life was when he shaved his head on my birthday, to match my bald head. Anything for his birthday girl.

CHILDHOOD

The year was 1980 and the place was Tiruchirappalli, the town where I grew up in India.

We were playing a trust game, wherein a bunch of teenagers catch young kids when they jump. A very simple act. It was an easy game for the younger kids as they trusted and adored the teenagers.

My sister yelled, "On the count of three, jump!"

"Yes," I squealed happily.

On the count of three, I jumped, flying high, directly toward my sister's arms, hoping she would catch me. My sister tried to catch me but unfortunately, I was way off the mark and hit the front gate with my head. Rumor has it that I cried—well, who wouldn't?

I was always the tomboy of the family and very mischievous. Often, when I was home, I was busy climbing the doors and windows around our house.

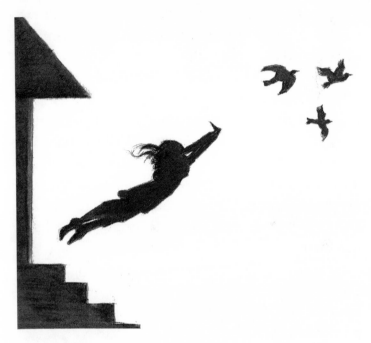

I never shrugged off doing anything adventurous. My five-year-old self was very sure that I could fly and the trust in my sister boosted my confidence. When I hit the gate, my sister rushed home to tell our mother. They hurried me to a clinic nearby. The doctor treated me with a few stitches to the forehead, the mark of which still resides on my forehead today. Per my sister, I was a brave little girl even then.

On the count of three, I tried to fly that day. But in my mind, I was always this little person who could fly, who could face any demon—well, any demon except cats. Cats, I was and am still afraid of. It is interesting to note the twists and turns that life takes. Does it treat you well or does life take you for granted? Does it provide you with ups and downs or does life let you be? Life surely shows most people how to deal with cats, but disease demands more from us.

SISTERLY LOVE

I was rebellious but generally honest; I did not mind a white lie every now and then to get away with skipping pills, to steal my sister's water colors, or to feign sickness to skip school. I was ready to do anything to follow in my sister's footsteps. Sometimes, taking it too literally and following her like a puppy. Hema, my second sister, was everything I was not. Seven years older than me, she was fair and beautiful, witty, and liked by all. I was dark, lanky, always walking around with a scowl on my face. She was what I wanted to grow up to be. She was my protector, warding off all evils but also my tormentor, the master who made me run her errands—some as simple as fetching water. One can always afford to be lazy with a starry-eyed little sister around to do your chores. She was pretty much the definition of a big sister, assiduously working for my progress while tormenting me with little stuff.

My eldest sister Uma, eleven years older, was out of our house by the time I was five years old and has always been more like a visitor in my memory. More of a maternal figure than a sister. The kind of sister who loved you like a mother. The one who you are forced to listen to, whether you agree or not. The sister who is touted as a role model and the one you strive to emulate. The sister whose visits you look forward to and expect gifts.

VITILIGO

A few months after my fall, I was diagnosed with vitiligo. It is a disorder where you get white patches on your skin due to melanin deficiency. Nothing life-threatening but not a good sight to see. Especially for a dark-skinned girl growing up in the 80s in India. Many Indians in those days, and some even today, considered white or at least light brown skin as the favored color for a person to look beautiful. As racist as that thinking seems, it was true then and, for some people, the belief remains deeply embedded today.

Imagine the plight of parents who have a dark-skinned daughter with white patches. They were worried about my future and immediately decided to find a good doctor who could cure me of the disorder.

My ever-loving father took me to various doctors after consulting his friends; he would not rest until he found a solution. We visited various doctors practicing different types of medicines, including allopathy, medicine as we know it, what we use in our day-to-day life; alternative medicines like homeopathy, treatment of disease by using tiny doses of liquidated natural substances; and Ayurveda, and Siddha, which is practiced mostly in South India, consisting of a mixture of herbs and sometimes metals.

One evening, when I was in the first grade, my dad came to the school to pick me up and shuttle me to a doctor in Tanjore, a town an hour away from Tiruchirappalli, the city where we lived. Since I hated these doctor visits with a passion, I intentionally hid from my father to avoid going with him to the doctor. Instead, I went home in the school rickshaw. Rickshaws were very common in India in those days. It is a vehicle pulled or pedaled by humans with seats for passengers. Schools were filled with rickshaws and groups of students were shuttled from home to school and back by rickshaw-wallah, the person pedaling the rickshaw.

Sure enough, after I reached home, my anxious father showed up to take me to the doctor. I was very confident that I had dodged that visit by hiding from dad at school. Alas, life doesn't always grant your wishes so easily. It takes its own time. I learned my first lesson that day. Running or hiding from struggles and dislikes does not make them go away. They always come back to find you, just like my father found me. His intentions were noble, out of pure love for me, and the trip to the doctor essential. Who knows what one might learn when facing struggles instead of running away from them? I suppose I was not destined to wait too long to learn how to face struggles.

We did finally end up visiting that doctor and he treated me for a few months with some pills and tablets. As a child, I could go one full day without food, but no one could ever make me swallow a pill. My throat could distinguish between a pill versus a grape and refused to gulp it down. I had a clear-cut plan to help my throat: take the pill from mom with a smile, pause slowly, go out, throw the pill out the window, and gulp the water down. This went on until the day my sister found the pills under the windowsill. The throwing was promptly reported to mom, and I was let go with some spanking and strict warnings. I did not realize then that this punishment came from their concern and best intentions for me. I hated gulping the pills with every cell in my body.

Even more disheartening was the complementary treatment: I was asked to stand naked facing the sun, with only my underwear on, every morning for ten minutes. For a self-conscious six-year-old, it was not easy, especially since we did not have a backyard and lived in a colony of houses. So, I had to stand outside the house. The plan was UV therapy for vitiligo. All I remember is the shame and self-consciousness of how others would perceive this. The day always started with this act. Retrospectively, it doesn't seem to be that awful for a six-year-old to stand naked, especially when the whole world is busy inside their houses getting ready for the day. But, at the time, it was one more difficult pill to swallow.

That remedy did not work and luckily for me, dad found a Siddha specialist (a doctor providing alternate herbal remedies) near home who was known for curing various disorders. No more standing in the sun. I was not worried about not getting cured of vitiligo but instead rejoiced that there were no more long trips or standing in the sun.

PRIMARY SCHOOL

"Shoba, what is the white patch on your eyelid?"

"Will it go away?"

"You look very weird."

Although some things changed for the better, the kids at school were a source of dismay. Classmates taunted me and were afraid to sit next to me due to the stigma attached to vitiligo. Kids see only what they see at face value. Unfortunately, they are brutally honest too. Many refused to play with me. I felt ashamed and unmotivated for many days, but I sustained my belief that my doctor and my dad would cure me.

Every morning and night, I religiously took my medicine, which was a mixture of herbs. During my childhood there were other priorities like exams, friends, festivals, holidays and so, the thought of how my vitiligo could affect my future never occurred to me. I had a very supportive family and a fine set of friends who helped me to show my friendly confidence, my brave will power, and my happy-go-lucky persona.

Taking siddha medications comes with lot of dietary restrictions and I was asked to follow it strictly for maximum benefit. I was not allowed to eat many vegetables including potatoes, tomatoes, and eggplant to name a few. Seriously, who in their right mind can forego potatoes—the one tuber universally loved by the whole world in various forms?

I did not mind the diet restrictions but hated other concoctions that I was forced to ingest. Lots of greens. I doubt if there is a six-year-old in the world, who would agree to load on greens and not eat potatoes. But everyone in the family watched me like a hawk and ensured a potato or tomato never reached my stomach.

Despite mother's consistent attention to my physical needs, my handsome, loving father was always my role model. He emulated what he preached. He loved community service and encouraged positivity. His daughters' education was his ultimate priority in life, and he worked very hard for that, not splurging on anything for himself. Seeing his daughter with a disorder nearly broke him. He searched far and near until he hit upon the best doctor to treat my vitiligo.

BUILDING MEMORIES WITH FATHER

"Get ready. We will be going to the doctor in the evening," I was told.

"Oh no!" I cried.

My parents were very diligent about my monthly visit to the doctor for my vitiligo as they were seeing some improvements. Some of my white patches were turning darker miraculously. With darker patches, my sunny disposition became even sunnier. Thanks to the Siddha doctor and his herbal medications, my vitiligo was cured successfully over fifteen years, except for a few lingering patches on my knees.

One night, my father took me to the doctor on his bicycle. It was a three-kilometer ride. Dad always used his bicycle as the mode of transport. For work, he was chauffeured in a car and hence never needed a vehicle as we used public transport to go everywhere. At the

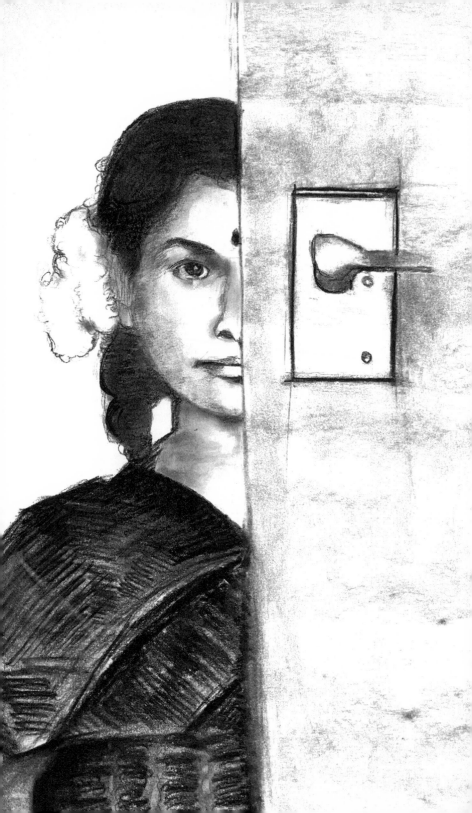

doctor's office, there was the usual examination where he checked out the progress of the patches and gave me the herbal medicine. There was always a treat at the end of the exam. Though the treat was just a couple of candies, it was always the high note of the day.

That night though, I was in for a marvelous surprise. My father rode his bicycle to the cinema theatre instead of going back home. Of course, my mother was part of the whole charade. My special treat! That night, I saw the biggest dog in the world. We watched the movie *Digby, the Biggest Dog in the World*. The movie-goers saw a beaming kid proud of her dad, full of adoration, looking at him with eyes brimming with love when we walked out of the theater. We came back home to be welcomed with a hot dinner from mother.

My father loved watching movies, while topping it off with good food. Every weekend, we were guaranteed a movie and a dinner. It was a custom that was followed in the Rao household for quite a while. We could be happy, sad, calm, or stressed, but the dinner tradition stayed alive. He introduced us to Hollywood movies, and we enjoyed every one of them though they took eons to reach India. We watched *Digby, the Biggest Dog in the World* ten years after it was released.

My father loved surprising us and that never stopped. When I was working at Texas Instruments, one evening, he called me and asked me to come to the theater. The internet was still not prevalent, and I had no idea what he was up to. There he was, standing with two tickets to *GoldenEye,* a movie with Pierce Brosnan as Bond, James Bond.

Father was as sensitive as he was brave. When I was in my second year of college, some major riots were brewing because the chief minister of the state we were living in India went on a hunger strike. Lots of drama to gain attention. Without any knowledge of the riots brewing, I hopped onto the bus going to the college town, which was a mere 150 km away. Everything looked hunky dory when I boarded the bus early in the morning. But, halfway through, the bus got stopped by some rioters and they refused to let the bus go, making us disembark. Luckily, one gentleman in the bus saw my plight, a young girl who was all alone and offered to help. When his boss came to pick him up, they offered to give me a ride to the nearest town where their office was located.

This was an era with no cellphone and there was no way I could reach my dad as we did not have a phone in our house either. When I finally got hold of the phone and was able to reach Dad, he was panicking and had started searching for me as soon as he heard the riots. A crying dad ran to hug me, and the driver said, "I have never seen your father crying before. He is such a brave man". He was brave indeed. It was the same brave man who lovingly took off from work when I was down with the measles, just so he could help carry me back and forth from the bathroom.

2 College Days
Courage And Determination

"OH! NO! Who will braid my hair tomorrow?"

"Shoba, Mom is in hospital and all you are worried about is your hair?" my sister lamented.

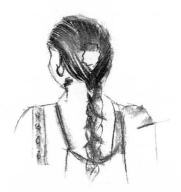 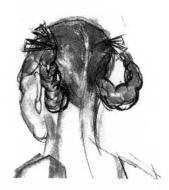

NAIVETY

When you are eleven years old, your priorities are different. You must ensure that someone takes you to school, your hair is not messy, your uniform is washed and pressed, and your lunch is packed. My mother had been taken severely ill and was hospitalized the previous night. She was feeling unwell the whole day and collapsed in a heap, later in the night. We learned later that she was admitted because of arrhythmia. Her heart was skipping every beat after three beats. She has that condition still today, but it has not affected her life. We are not perfect, and I guess she could afford to be off beat every now and then.

But that day all I worried about was the sorrow my long locks would be feeling if not braided properly. The alarming question looming ahead was, "Who will braid my hair the next morning?" Sometimes, I wish I could revisit that eleven-year-old every now and then as I was always a happy-go-lucky girl. Nothing fazed me much and I went with the flow life showed me. Like many children that age, I was still self-absorbed enough to care about my braid when my mother was in a hospital bed.

Mother came back from the hospital after a few days and things started becoming normal again. My braids were as good as ever. I went on to finish my schooling at Thiruchirapalli, a small town in Tamil Nadu, a southern state in the Indian subcontinent.

Having two sisters who were accomplished in whatever they pursued placed a lot of extra pressure on my tiny shoulders. My eldest sister, Uma, was a gold medalist in her B.E. (bachelor of engineering) degree and was pursuing her master's in electrical engineering while working as a lecturer. My second sister, Hema, was also pursuing her B.E. in electrical engineering. Everyone expected me to be as competent as them, if not more.

MY PERFORMANCE

Even as a child, I realized that the best way to handle any pressure is to brush it off as trivial and work hard to ensure people have as low an expectation as possible from you. Once the baseline is set, there is no way but upwards; you will appear accomplished with everyone

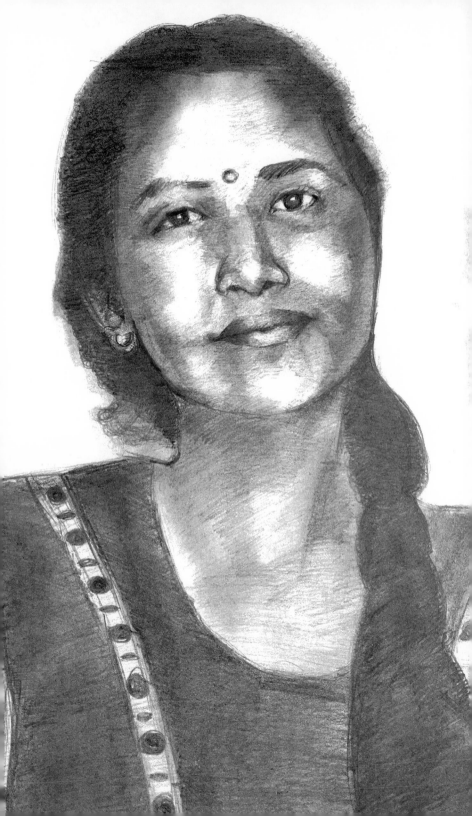

praising you for your effort and participation. I was always a rebel and made sure nothing and no one pushed me to do something I did not want to do. That said, my schooling did end, and I passed with flying colors—maybe just a couple shades short of the full spectrum, but enough to satisfy myself and others.

My father never had high hopes for me as I rarely worked hard to score better marks. My photographic memory helped me achieve good grades and be in the top 5% of my class. Having the "memory of an elephant" carried me all the way through my undergraduate degree with a Bachelor of Engineering at a school in Erode, a neighboring city.

My college was conservative, like many in southern India in the 90s. We had to be always dressed in traditional Indian attire. My rebellious streak whispered to me to immediately quit and move to another college. But I prevailed. The four years spent in Erode, away from my parents, surrounded by strangers who later I called my friends, taught me more than what I had learned in my entire lifetime until then.

There was a lot of ragging by seniors, and I was a consistent target for many, slowly building the reputation as someone who was too strong and arrogant. Ragging is a fun practice wherein the senior students get an excuse to harass their junior counterparts. Rebel that I was, I remained motivated despite the constant ragging. Those four years taught me how to navigate in life and manage friends and foes alike. This is where life presented me with some of my best friends and my best friend forever,

Suresh. When anyone asks if I regret attending a medio-
cre college for my Bachelor of Engineering, I always say,
"Never. That is where I made some great friends and
where I met Suresh, the strongest pillar in my life. My
own Samurai who is always with me."

REVELATION

College is where I learned an important lesson: Because I
acted like a spoiled brat whose grades came easily to her,
I was arrogant and stubborn. I never apologized or yielded
to others much, except maybe some close friends. One fine
morning, while visiting home, my eldest sister Uma gave
me a piece of her mind when I was in one of my moods
of being cranky, stubborn, and aggressive. She said that
there would come a time when no one would want to talk
to me or be with me if I continued my behavior, and that
I would be an embarrassment to my parents. Those were
very harsh words spoken but very true as well. I needed
to hear what she had to say as I consider that day to be a
turning point in my life; I intentionally started to work on
changing myself. It was not easy but taking one step at a
time, I was determined to achieve that.

My four years in college were a mixture of good and
bad moments, ups and downs typical to what life usually teaches you. Life is like a roller coaster ride with
your friends with some emotional moments, some fun
moments, some naughty, some frustrating, some san-
guine, and some melodramatic. Ah, the life of a college
student. I am glad I passed it with flying colors and formed
some marvelous friendships that I cherish to date.

COURAGE AND DETERMINATION

Though I was happy-go-lucky, I was brave and determined when the occasion demanded. Bullying by others never affected me. I have been bullied countless times by other students, especially boys. Once, there was a misunderstanding among the guys that I had belittled one of their mates. He was another student in my class, and my roommate's younger brother added some fuel to curry favors from the boys—a childish gesture from a spoiled kid. Unfortunately, it became a big issue, and I was swarmed by angry guys from various departments asking for explanations for which I had none as I had no clue what they were talking about. It took a lot of effort to look brave, let alone stand my ground in front of those angry young men.

I was equally determined not to let my friends get bullied. During our final year in college, one of my friends studying in a field where she was the only girl in her class got bullied by all the boys in her class and came back to the hostel crying. Not taking it lying down, an entourage of four girls, led by Susheela, my best friend and I, walked over to the campus and confronted the key harasser. Surrounded by four angry girls made him shrink and say that he was sorry. That is what we were made of: loyal to friends and ready to face any fight for them.

Other than my sleep-enhanced elephant's memory, it was these strengths—courage and determination—that carried me forward through my college years. As things turned out, this same courage and determination were going to sustain me through some very trying times in the years ahead.

3 Why Me, Why Now?

Listen To Your Body

"ARE WE THERE YET?" I asked.

"Just a few more steps, we should reach the summit soon," my friend encouraged.

My friends were encouraging me to climb farther. At least, that's what I wanted to believe though they might have not wanted a weak link on their hike. There must be a weak link in every climb and every group, and that day, I was the weakest. Some of my friends from Texas Instruments, where I was working at the time, decided to hike a mountain near a colleague's house. In all my naivete, I decided to toughen myself and climb with them.

LISTEN TO YOUR BODY

Halfway through the climb, I realized that I was totally out of shape and hence out of breath. It reminded me of the novel, *The Goal* by Eliyahi Goldratt. In the novel, Goldratt lays out what he terms a "theory of constraints." The idea is that the success of an entire factory (or, in fact, of any process at all) is determined by the choke point that constrains the overall output. But whatever the bottleneck is, every action should be taken with it in mind, and every resource should be directed at eliminating it. Once the worst bottleneck is identified and vaporized, you go hunting for the next worst, and then the next.[1]

On that day, I was the choke point in our climb.

Fortunately, my friends had not read the book and did not think of eliminating the bottleneck. The whole climb slowed down with everyone stopping for me, every few yards. I worried that something was seriously wrong with me.

BLOOD TESTS

As soon as I came back home, I shared my worries with my parents and sister. Since the family had already been through some health hurdles with father's heart bypass surgery, we were well-informed when it came to the novelty of blood tests and the human body. As a family, it was decided to test my hemoglobin. Hemoglobin (Hb) is a protein found in the red blood cells that carries oxygen in your body and gives blood its red color.

In India, you don't need a doctor's prescription or order to take a blood test. You pay and let the clinician know what you are looking for. A prick never mattered to me though I was yet not used to the poking and pricking that would come later. The blood test came back with an Hb count of 6.0. A low hemoglobin count is generally defined as less than 13.5 grams of hemoglobin per deciliter (135 grams per liter) of blood for men and less than 12 grams per deciliter (120 grams per liter) for women. On a scale of one to ten for normalcy, my value was a zero. Now, there was the reason for being the weakest link on my hike. It was not me; it was my red blood cell count.

We decided to visit a primary care doctor near our house. The doctor we went to was astonished to see me walking around instead of falling in a slump. I had even

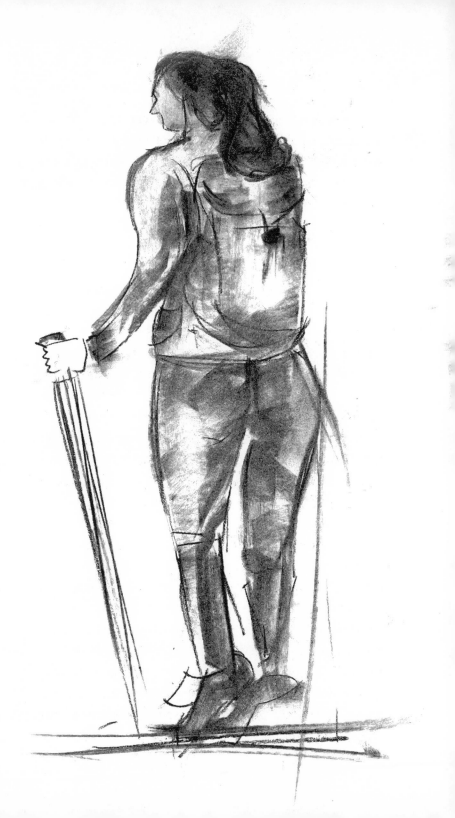

won a mixed double table tennis (TT) tournament just a few weeks back at work. It was a mystery to all of us. Apparently, my body was more resilient than I gave it credit for and molded itself to my mental strength. It was helping me survive, with a win in a TT tournament thrown in for good measure.

THE IMPORTANCE OF IRON

After scratching his head a few times and marveling at my magical strength, the doctor decided to start me on some iron tablets to boost my Hb.

My mother, not to be outdone, introduced a diet full of iron every day. If there was anyone in this wide world who knew how to take care of me with food, that would be my mother. I consumed dates soaked in honey every single day. I had spinach and other greens pureed, steamed, baked, hidden in some form or other in every dish I ate. With the dates working their magic, one month later, I was tested for Hb levels again. It turned out to be more of a decline than a progression. Not exactly what we were aiming for. My Hb went down from 6.0 to 5.0. Apparently, my body decided to be resilient in fighting the iron tablets too. Not one to give up a fight, my doctor started pumping me with iron injections every week.

After coming back from work, every week, father and I used to walk to the clinic. The doctor administered the painful injections, with me bravely walking back home with all the pain radiating down my leg due to the injections. Coming home invariably ended with me throwing up, clearing my stomach even if it was just bile fluid. During the process, my whole wish was that a few throw ups and toss ups did not matter if I could work up my hemoglobin.

After one more month, when tested again, unfortunately, the level did not come up, and I was back to square one. This finally alarmed the doctor and he referred me for a full blood test and scan, while also referring me to his friend at a well-known hospital. There started the anxious journey of scans, blood tests and the whole shebang. I told a few of my friends at work about the situation, the kind of colleagues with who I could share my anxiety though it sounded like Greek or Latin to them.

BLOOD TRANSFUSIONS

I was pumped with some blood as the first line of treatment for bringing up my Hb, while waiting for my scan results. My uncle and brother-in-law generously donated blood for me. Those were the first pints of external blood that went into my body. Ah, the acrobatics one must do to up the hemoglobin count. Although I was turning rosy after the blood pumping, my scans and results were not that rosy. Apparently, both my kidneys had shrunk to half their size and my creatinine level was at 3.0.

Creatinine is a chemical waste product that's produced by your muscle metabolism and to a smaller extent by eating meat. Healthy kidneys filter creatinine and other waste products from your blood. If your kidneys aren't functioning properly, an increased level of creatinine may accumulate in your blood. The normal range for creatinine in the blood may be 0.84 to 1.21

milligrams per deciliter. Mine was at 3.0 mg. Generally, it feels good to be high, but being high in creatinine was not really helping me. The nephrologist, a kidney specialist, from the hospital I was admitted to, walked into my room, nodded his head gravely and announced that I had chronic renal failure. I had no clue what that meant except that it sounded grave, maybe one step closer to the grave. I nodded my head gravely too. And then cried. My parents had no clue either, but I could sense the fright in their faces. My mother, with tears brimming in her eyes, looked at me and said, "Don't worry, Shoba. I am here and will take care of you". I was crying too, not knowing what renal failure meant though I knew it sounded fatal.

The nephrologist who diagnosed me did not have a great bedside manner. He was very blunt and rude in the way he told us about the diagnosis. He took my father aside and drew a graph showing how long it would be before I die, all the while consoling him. "You have two more daughters to look forward to, Mr. Keshava Rao, even if one were to kick the bucket". Yes, he assumed that would soothe my dad's pain. The graph had the number of years on the x-axis and kidney function on the y-axis, with the kidney deteriorating over a few years resulting in my death. My father is a stoic, sensitive and loving man who faced all the hurdles life threw at him and worked hard to protect and educate his daughters. Though his heart was full of worry, he tried not to show it to others. But we all could feel the big black elephant in the room.

KIDNEY FAILURE

Chronic renal failure (CRF), in layman's terms, means kidney failure. It was as mundane as that. It was chronic because it happened over time, slowly creeping in. The cause of my kidney failure was not known and one that none of us could fathom. I don't think I ever grasped the seriousness of the disease until the day I saw my dad talking to one of his cousins, Ravi, who had stopped by to enquire about my health. I was in my room, behind a curtain and saw my dad with a helpless expression, telling Ravi, "It's all over. I am not sure how long she will survive."

I felt like a huge burden to my parents. The gravity of the situation hit me—literally and figuratively. I had to lie down for a while to absorb it all. Though my dad felt like it was doomsday, he was not ready to give in that easily and immediately started looking for options. We went to various hospitals, who did the same scans and blood tests and always came back with the same diagnosis. "There is no cure other than dialysis." I vividly remember the day when we came back from Madras, a different city than the one I lived in, where we had visited Tamil Nadu hospital. I walked into my cubicle at work and one of my colleagues was waiting eagerly to know the results and find out if we had found a cure. I looked at him with a blank face and said, "That's it man! I am done. The doctors have all given up." No tears, no sorrow, and no feelings. Interestingly, no fear too. Only anguish. Anguish that I may not be able to experience life with all its beauty and color. I was thinking about it constantly at work and walking around like a zombie.

I even called a couple of very good friends of mine and told them goodbye as I sincerely thought I was done with life. Rather, life was done with me. It was obvious it did not want me around anymore. More than the question of "Why me?" my question was "Why now?" Why not when I was young enough not to understand what was happening. Why not later in life when I would've been older and wiser with a successful career, ready to accept kidney failure. A nice wedding and marriage to some handsome young man would have been a bonus. Instead, it was just a couple of years into my career, and I had to face the pursuit of a cure.

A NEW NEPHROLOGIST

Finally, my father found a nephrologist who had a track record of successful kidney transplants, at The Lakeside Memorial Hospital in Bangalore. Dr. Sundar was a very charming, confident, and sensitive nephrologist. There was a transplant team in the hospital and for the era of 1997, they had already done numerous transplants. Meeting Dr. Sundar boosted my confidence. He was my savior, someone who gave me the confidence that I could be cured someday. He was a logical, pragmatic, kind-hearted and sympathetic doctor who did not mince words while being very compassionate and reassuring.

Kidney disease must be taken care of with major dietary restrictions. I couldn't eat much protein, salt, fruits, potassium rich vegetables, or drink more than three cups of water per day. The preferred way to eat vegetables was to fully boil them, removing all the nutrients as much as possible prior to eating them. With my already low weight, adding the exceptionally restrictive diet, I reached a new low of thirty-seven kgs (eighty-two pounds). Light as a feather.

HOMEOPATHY

Meanwhile, my sister suggested a homeopathic doctor who supposedly had magic hands with a proven track record. We went to meet him as a family. While noting down my whole history, one of his questions stood out, "Have you ever fallen as a child?" We had no idea why that was asked, but indeed I had fallen from a reasonable height as a six-month old child.

As humans, when faced with a life and death scenario, the logical brain wants to understand the reason. As if knowing the reason would change everything. But the question exists, "Why, oh why?" My sister and mother recounted the whole incident of my fall as a six-month-old, and we decided to latch onto it. Finally, it felt like we had the answer to the "why" question. Though we latched on to the fall, we realized shortly that the fall had nothing to do with kidney failure.

My monthly visit to Dr. Rampriya, the homeopathy doctor, was a chore. I traveled in my company's bus for one hour, then caught a taxi to the doctor's office. My dad came to the doctor's office in a bus, and we took a taxi back, reaching home by 10 p.m. Mother anxiously waited for us to learn if there was any progress. Despite all the treatments, my creatinine had slowly crept up from 3.0 to 5.0. It was very disheartening to do so much work and still end up getting even worse.

Sometimes, I stayed at my sister's house which was near the doctor's clinic. On one such night, when I caught an auto to go to the clinic, one of my friends from work also hopped in, much to my surprise. He had sensed something was wrong with me and wanted to find out about my mysterious visits every week. Much to his chagrin, I was brushing it all off and making fun of everything. He had gotten into the auto to find out where I was going. When I told him that I had kidney failure, his eyes started filling up and in a choked voice, he said, "I am angry at God." Yes, I was angry at God. Why me? Why now?

4 Kidney Transplant
Don't Let Your Struggles Stop You From Living

"SHOBA, I THINK it's better to get your fistula surgery done and prepare you for dialysis."

"What is a fistula, Doc?" I asked, making a fist assuming it had to do something with my palms. Maybe an 'ula' was the size of my fist, but I was sure he would tell me what 'ula' really meant.

"We create a path for a stronger and faster blood flow in your veins, by connecting your artery and vein near your wrist. That vein will be used for dialysis as the vein will be able to tolerate thicker needles since its walls would have become thicker due to the high arterial pressure."

DIALYSIS PREP
All I heard was pressure and veins and that some surgery had to be done. It sounded vague and indistinct. Not the definition I was hoping for. My arm had to be operated upon to get it ready for dialysis, in plain English.

First and foremost, Dr. Sundar accepted that he doesn't know the cause of my kidney failure while also advising me to stop taking my vitiligo medicine, a mixture of herbs that I had been consuming for fifteen years. He suspected that the herbs could have been the cause, but there was no way to prove it. I still remember his phrase, "If a medicine has effects, there will always be side effects, too. Natural herbs are not the equivalent of harmless". Though he did not have much faith in natural herbs, he did not steer me away from my homeopathy medicine that I had been taking to cure my kidney failure. He did not want me to lose faith. However, he asked me to be prepared for emergency dialysis while trying homeopathy drugs to cure my kidney failure.

That was the beginning of my interaction with surgeons and surgeries. The arteriovenous (AV) fistula surgery is very simple and was performed by one of the junior doctors at the hospital. I stayed overnight at the hospital as I was very anemic. Two of my friends donated blood to get me out of the woods that day.

B-positive (B+) is the most common blood group in India, next only to O+, which helped the cause as every other friend of mine was positive that he was B+. Thank God that I could be positive about being B+. That night, I developed a very high fever, and my mother was next to my bed through the night, her presence helping to alleviate my pain. I often wonder what mothers are made of, to always be there when you need them.

The next day, I was discharged and went to work as usual. Except for a selected few very close friends and important managers, no one knew about my medical conditions. I never showed any symptoms of going through a slow kidney failure process.

DON'T LET YOUR STRUGGLES
STOP YOU FROM LIVING

I continued my homeopathy treatments for five more months with no cure in sight. My mother insisted that

I go ahead with the kidney transplant as soon as possible, especially because she would rather have a surgery at fifty-four years old than later. In the hospital when I was diagnosed with kidney failure, my mother had said she would do whatever it took to save me. True to those words, as soon as she learned that a transplant could save my life, she immediately volunteered to donate one of her kidneys to give me a second chance at life. My mother was petrified of surgeries. Camouflaging her fear, she got ready for the transplant. She had to go through a renal angiography to make decisions on which kidney to transplant. It was decided that the left kidney was going to be the hero and my savior. We both were admitted to the hospital a couple of days before the day of the surgery. My eldest sister, Uma, who was living in another state, traveled to Bangalore to help us for a month after the surgery. She was my go-to person for all issues during that period; someone with a maternal instinct who guided me along and the one who I relied upon.

I never let my struggles affect me. One of my colleagues always used to wonder how I am happy most of the time. One fine morning when I was in the elevator on the way to my floor at work, three of my colleagues walked in. One, who knew my health hurdles and two others who were unaware. K., who was clueless about my condition, asked "How is life?" "Pretty good," I replied. Nodding at G., who knew I had just had my surgery, K. said, "Our lives are never fine. What is so special about Shoba's life that it is always pretty good." G. nodded with an awkward smile. But my life was pretty good after all. I was prepared for emergency dialysis, trying homeopathy drugs, and would receive my wonderful mother's kidney to save my life. What else could one ask for in life?

I wanted to lead my life as normally as possible. The fact that most of my colleagues were unaware of my condition helped me immensely. I went to work without a break until the day before the transplant. The day before the transplant, and after work, when I walked into the hospital, my niece Arathi, Uma's daughter, ran over to me and gave me a hug. One of those welcome, delightful hugs which only an innocent child can give. She has always been my most favorite child since she was born. She was just nine years old then but cared about me so much that she even offered to donate her kidney when she learned that her blood group was B positive, same as mine. As someone who was constantly around her elders, she had decided that kidney failure was lethal, and it was of supreme importance for me to get a kidney.

This was a very sweet and generous gesture from a child, especially one who very rarely was willing to share her goodies. On that day, when Arathi and I were playing in the hospital, I noticed an elderly gentleman observing us from afar. He walked over and asked if I was visiting someone and how the patient was doing. That whole wing in the hospital was only for transplant patients. He peeped into the room vaguely and noticed my mother sitting in the hospital bed. On his questioning further about my mother, I explained that I was the patient with kidney failure and my mother was the donor. He was flabbergasted and speechless as he could not fathom that a transplant patient could be enjoying herself the day before surgery as though there was not a care in the world.

He was there at the hospital to visit and take care of his son-in-law who was extremely depressed and had had a transplant the previous day. Seeing me brightened his day and I became his hero from that moment. His adoration and love became almost embarrassing when he brought all their visitors for a show-and-tell in our room for the next whole week.

I was anything but inspiring. My fears were well-concealed by a façade of strength and bravery. My young age and the huge support system among my friends and family helped me cope with my fears and negative thoughts. We humans have an excellent, resilient system, and our brain is an amazing device with selective amnesia when needed. The same selective amnesia that makes you go for the chocolate cake when you know it is unhealthy for you. You don't remember the unhealthy part, do you?

TRANSPLANT SURGERY

There was enough positive energy around me to assist me in forgetting my fear and to go through the surgery as yet another simple process as if to say, "I have been there and done that." My whole family, with an entourage of uncles and aunts, were at the hospital on the day of the surgery. My colleagues from Texas Instruments, especially my boss and dear friends, were outside the operating theater until I was wheeled out. Word has it that they skipped lunch as they were too worried about how I would fare and were waiting patiently until the surgery was done.

As often happens in life, things do not always go ahead smoothly. My surgery reached a crisis at the operating table, when suddenly, the doctors said they could not do the surgery because of my mother's arrhythmia. They were not sure how her heart would handle the surgery since it was off beat. I was wheeled in, about to be administered local anesthesia, when I heard the doctors whispering about my mother.

Holy cow, oh no! No surgery? Fear kicked in and had me almost paralyzed. Luckily, at the last minute, the doctors decided to go ahead with the surgery. Both mother and I were operated on at the same time and her kidney was immediately transferred into my teeny tiny body—I weighed a mere thirty-eight kilograms then. They left my native kidneys intact as they were not infected. We all have our kidneys behind the rib cages at the back. The transplanted kidney is placed in the front, next to the bladder. During my many scans over the following years, many radiologists were thrilled when they saw the kidney at an unusual location. I suppose this is my service to humanity—making people happy in small ways.

A left donor kidney is usually implanted on your right side; a right donor kidney implanted on your left side. My mother's kidney was implanted in the right side of my abdomen. This allows the ureter to be accessed easily for connection to your bladder. The renal artery and vein of her kidney were sewn to the external iliac artery and vein. The ureter (the tube that drains urine from the kidney) of her kidney was connected to my bladder. Sounds simple enough, and was, thanks to my surgeon.

HOW DID WE DO?

As soon as I came out of sedation in the operation room, my first question was to check how mother was faring as the last thing I had heard before falling asleep was about mother's arrhythmia. I was not given a full anesthesia, but instead was given a local anesthesia in my spine, similar to an epidural which paralyzed me from my thighs down. Imagine regaining your consciousness and realizing that you cannot move your legs. Despite being still under sedation a bit, my panic showed in my voice when I started shouting that I could not move my legs. I am sure though I was shouting, it might have sounded more like murmuring to the doctors. Well, most often in India, unfortunately or fortunately, the doctors don't tell you much and they did not prepare me with what to expect. But they were patient enough to answer all my questions when I was wheeled out of the surgery and into the ICU.

The surgery was a success and both mother and I were sent home just after a week. My mother was healing well along with me. I was taking regular walks in the hospital before the discharge. The amazing support from my family showed in myriad ways: my paternal Uncle Bhavani Shankar brought breakfast from his house every morning and my Aunt Teju, cousin Sudha, and friends assisted in various ways by staying at the hospital. Of course, my father and sisters were always there by our side.

After reaching home, I realized that a transplant surgery involves more than just going under the knife. The
follow-up medicines take a toll on you and your wallet. For
the surgery, my savings along with money loaned from
my employer covered all the costs. The medicines after
the transplant were very expensive and my insurance was
not covering them. I had to consume ten tablets/capsules
every day. Luckily, I earned enough to cover those expenses
as boarding and lodging were free, the perk of staying with
parents. I was under strict advice not to venture out for
two months without wearing a mask; the immunosup-
pressive drugs that are given to ensure the new kidney did
not get rejected, were bringing my immunity way down,
making me susceptible to infections.

5 Life Post-Transplant
Keep Working And Moving On

"YOU CAN EAT whatever you want," the doctor said.

Additionally, he emphasized, "Just ensure you don't go to crowded places."

NEW LOVE OF FOOD

The doctors sent me home with those words and that is when my love for food started. This was a temptation of the unknown because until my transplant, I was not able to eat much and was constantly nauseated. After my surgery, I started enjoying and relishing every single morsel.

My sister Uma helped both me and my mom recuperate and recover. She took time off from her busy schedule, staying with us at Bangalore just to ensure both her mother and her sister recovered fully. If there was one other person in the family who is adept at facing hurdles like a pro, that would be my darling sister Uma. She doesn't get fazed very easily even though she has her own set of health issues to battle. She even flew to California to support me during one of my chemo journeys.

I gained a few pounds not just because of the steroids but also due to my intake of ample food, much to my mother's delight. Getting a transplant gave me a new lease of life. The burst of energy and the ability to eat good food without feeling nauseated was as refreshing as standing under a waterfall. A waterfall of renewed energy and new medicines. I was able to feel and enjoy life with fresh eyes. The mask was the only hindrance.

DON'T LET YOUR STRUGGLES DICTATE YOUR LIFE

Other than food, the most important item on my agenda was hygiene and protecting my immune system. Doctors had advised me to wear a mask most of the time when interacting with outsiders and at work. I was wearing a mask when we had visitors, when I went for my early morning walk, when I had to do some work around the house, and even when there was nobody around me. Being in India with its one billion population, it was not easy to walk in a public park avoiding eye contact with people you know because even a glance in that direction ensures a follow up smile with the person slowly walking towards you. With the mask, very few recognized me anyway and having time to myself was not too tough. Imagine going to a party only to be told you cannot greet others and must sit in one corner quietly.

The doctors had given me three months to recuperate before going back to work. Three months sounded like a very long time, and I decided to use it effectively by learning how to drive. Retrospectively, I am not sure what I was thinking. Sometimes, foolishness is camouflaged as bravery. This would have been an excellent example. Learning to drive in a crowded metro like Bangalore, with smokes/fumes everywhere while recovering from a transplant surgery was the height of foolishness. My brain assumed the mask to be made of iron and just went along with what the heart said. Learning and passing a driving test is almost child's play in India, a land where corruption is rampant, and bribery is the norm. I did not want to take the easy route and passionately wanted to learn driving. After all, until that time I had not learned to drive even a cycle and it was high time I knew how to go from one place to another on my own.

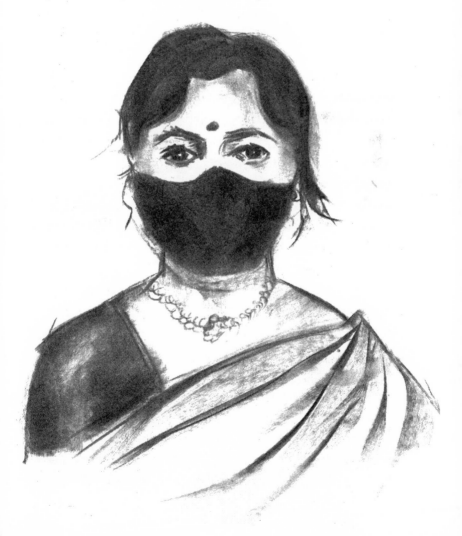

BACK TO WORK

After three months, I went back to work to a hilarious return as many of my colleagues were astounded seeing my face. The steroids had added at least fifteen pounds to my weight, and I was made more beautiful with a moon face due to prednisone. The ever-skinny Shoba had morphed into this moon-faced, plump woman. Though I was feeling a bit down about the moon face, I did perk up with the thought that I was alive. Who would not feel happy to receive an organ upon request from a parent, with all the stars perfectly aligned during the surgery? I will take living with a moon face any day in a heartbeat rather than suffering with dialysis. I did feel very uncomfortable initially when some people could not recognize me. Slowly it sunk in, and I became Shoba, Reinvented.

After my transplant, I was on a mission. A mission to live life my way and that being the only way. Life was short after all. I did not want to see the angry and sad faces surrounding me every day. I did not want to be pitied. Even going to work was making me feel suffocated.

Fortunately, just three months out of surgery and going back to work, a moon-faced woman who just learned to drive got the chance to go to the United States of America. My supervisors were a bit skeptical wondering how I could manage on my own in an unknown land with minimal support. Especially when it was only three months into my recovery. For someone who wanted to get away from it all, this was a golden opportunity. Nothing could stop me from grabbing the chance of a lifetime to get out of India, away from all the sad memories. To taste freedom. To be free—a luxury from my vantage point. By hook or by crook I was going, so I convinced everyone that I was definitely up to the challenge.

I landed in Dallas in November of 1998 with a lot of excitement and determination. The plan was to attend training and work for a few months. There were a couple of colleagues who were in the same apartment complex allocated to me, which helped with getting back and forth from work.

SURESH

One ray of hope to settle in easier was the knowledge that I had some friends from college living in the US, though not in Dallas. This included two close friends, Susheela in Los Angeles, and Suresh in San Jose, CA. I spent all my free time talking to them. Little did I know then that my life partner would be this bespectacled, lovely, loving, and benevolent gentleman, Suresh.

Our love blossomed slowly over time. Within a month after I landed in Dallas, Suresh flew from California to visit me. I did not have a driver's license yet, but badly wanted to travel around the US as I was very sure that I would not be able to come back after my tenure of a couple of months. When Suresh visited, I wanted him to take me around Texas. We drove and drove the whole day. We started from Dallas at 5:00 a.m., drove all the way to Houston, visited NASA Headquarters, drove to San Antonio from there as I wanted to visit Sea World. I had two goals while visiting the USA—one was seeing a dolphin and the other was playing in snow. I was eagerly looking forward to watching the dolphins swim at Sea World but unfortunately Sea World was closed for the winter.

Suresh enjoyed driving and was also an endearing friend who wanted to show me around. It was easy enough for him to drive back to Dallas via Austin. Overall, a drive of approximately one thousand miles in one day, before reaching Dallas at 2:30 a.m. That was the day I realized what happiness meant. What being carefree meant.

The next day at work, when my colleague asked about the weekend, I said, "I laughed and enjoyed myself after a long time. I had forgotten how good life felt until now." Retrospectively it is no surprise I ended up marrying this nice man. He came like a ray of sunshine into my life, making me feel protected and loved.

After that weekend, there were non-stop phone calls between Dallas and San Jose, despite the time difference. Every night, I went to sleep cradling the phone after a couple of hours of talking with Suresh. Friendship and camaraderie blossomed into love without our knowledge. I started viewing life differently. The added bonus was the extension of my stay to six months in Dallas, giving us more time to get to know each other. By the end of my six months stay, the proposal happened. I fell even more in love with that man and was ready to marry him.

Even today, whenever I see him, I fall in love again and again. I always wonder how the universe has been taking care of me, in the form of loving parents and sisters and in the form of the most benevolent man as a husband. I knew it was time to seal our love with a wedding vow.

After my six months stay was over, and I was back home, I informed my parents about our intentions.

MARRIAGE

My mother was thrilled as my marriage was weighing on her and she was constantly worried that I might never find a companion. My dad was a bit cautious but the fact that it was Suresh and not some random person I had met in the subway, helped him accept my decision. Interestingly, Suresh's parents also were totally fine with us getting married. They had already met me a couple of times when we were studying together, and this was not a shock. Our wedding date was finalized without any hassle.

In India, we have the concept of arranged marriages where often the families look for a bride or a groom for their sons and daughters. Once some basic needs are fulfilled and the family background is checked out with sometimes astrology thrown into the mix, the boy/girl starts filtering who he/she wants to marry. After meeting a few suitors, once it works out between two of them, the wedding is settled.

So, it was indeed a very pleasant surprise that both families agreed without hesitation. I flew back to the US to work again for six months and had the time of my life with Suresh. We used to meet each other almost every weekend as and when possible. Most often, Suresh flew from California to Dallas. The feeling of being in love, being adored with unconditional love is an experience I wish to happen for every living being in this world. We got married on January 23, 2000, with a lot of pomp and show.

Indian weddings go on and on with hundreds of people attending the wedding, that is full of fun and resplendent sarees, lehengas (long skirts) and dhotis (wrappers similar to a sarong).

MY CAREER

After the wedding, I moved to California the first week of February. Luckily, I had gotten my work visa on the day of the wedding and could make it to the US using my work visa instead of being a dependent. I was very adamant about not landing in a faraway country as a dependent. It was the result of values inculcated by my dad. He always emphasized that one must be independent and brave to face the world. I joined National Semiconductors as a senior engineer testing ADCs (Analog to Digital Converter). My career flourished there for four years until I moved to linear technology for a better opportunity. During those four years, other than gaining experience, I was able to take EE courses at Stanford, finish my GRE and get into the master's program at Stanford University.

On the health front, as soon as I landed in California, my first task was to find a good nephrologist. Thanks to my primary care provider, I found Dr. George Ting, a nephrologist who I have been seeing for the past twenty years. Dr. Ting is one of the most thorough physicians I have ever met in my life. He does not shrug off or ignore any of my symptoms or questions and monitors everything that is suspect.

He is a Godsend for me. He has been a key person in diagnosing my disorders and cancer at an early stage.

On my very first visit to Dr. Ting, he felt my neck and decided I had thyroid nodules and gave me a referral to an endocrinologist. I was surprised as no other doctor until then had ever suggested anything even remotely related to thyroid nodules. True to that, the ultrasound showed nodules in my thyroid, and I had the first biopsy of my life done on those nodules. It was a huge scare then as that was the first time, we ever heard anyone using the word cancer. The big "C" word that instills fear and doomsday. Luckily, the nodules turned out to be benign. Whew, a huge relief!

After my transplant surgery was completed and I came to the USA, I realized that taking prednisone (steroid) for too long comes with its own repercussions including blood pressure, lower bone density, diabetes, and high cholesterol. I was diagnosed with high blood pressure and osteopenia, a low bone density disorder. To the pile of current medications, in went Norvasc (blood pressure medication) and thyroxine for my thyroid nodules. From the little girl who threw medicines out of the window to the woman who was gobbling pills, I had come a long way, adding a little bit of wisdom, and acquiring additional acceptance of what life can bring into my character.

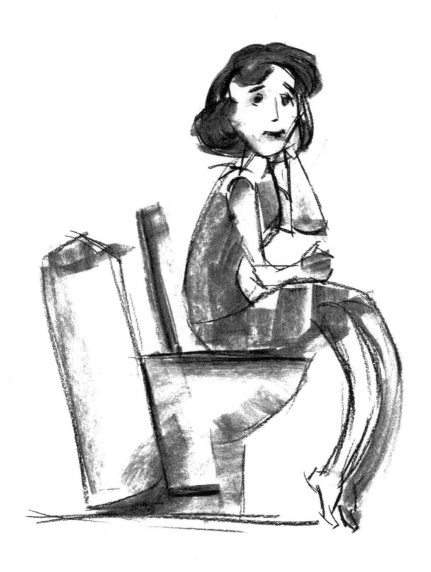

6 Cancer—The Beast
Be Positive. Brave It Through.

"I SAW BLOOD while peeing", I said gravely.

"Are you sure? Maybe, you got your periods."

My mind was reeling. Am I pregnant, by any chance? No way said the brain. Maybe, it was the stress, cried the heart as I was pursuing my M.S. in Electrical Engineering at Stanford University. I had to spend long nights finishing assignments and preparing for exams. I was halfway through my courses and wanted to finish my master's as soon as possible. Suresh had graduated the previous year (2003) and I was itching to catch up. We were just four years into our life together and still had a whole lifetime ahead. Blood in the urine was not exactly what I was looking for.

BLOOD IN MY URINE
November 2004 was the first time I ever saw blood in my urine. It didn't really alarm me. I thought I might have exerted myself a lot while working out. It did not alarm Suresh either as he was just catching up with all the medical jargon after our marriage. My nephrologist, Dr. Ting, was on vacation, and the attending doctor prescribed some antibiotics assuming it was an UTI (urinary tract infection). After ten days, the cranberry-colored urine alarmed me slightly.

Dr. Ting returned from vacation and ordered another urine culture test, which came out negative for bacteria but confirmed macroscopic and microscopic blood in my urine. I was very methodical so had the results of my ultrasound from a few months back ready in hand for the doctor to compare with my current ultrasound. He saw an obstruction/growth in my native right kidney

A few tense days were followed by a CT (computerized tomography) scan. That was the first CT scan in my life. To be honest, cancer was nowhere on my horizon then. I thought something was wrong with my kidney and was quite worried. The CT scan confirmed the blockage in my right ureter and Dr. Ting immediately put me in touch with a urologist, Dr. Aigen. A biopsy date was set up and I was scheduled to get one immediately.

A SILVER LINING AMIDST PAIN

After the biopsy procedure, I was in the recovery room until late at night as my pain level would not come down. It was painful to answer the nurse with a "ten" whenever she asked what my pain level was, with one for the least pain and ten for the most pain. The following few days were some of the most painful I have ever had in my life so far. The pain was due to the tumor blocking my ureter and the flow of urine. Unfathomable, unbearable pain. I was on codeine to combat the pain, which was not helping much except for a couple of hours after the medication was ingested.

At the same time, my last exam for that quarter was due. I could not risk going to Stanford because of the pain. Luckily, my professors honored the honor code and let me take the exam at home with Suresh monitoring. Interestingly, I got an A+ in that course, much to my elation. A cloud of silver lining amid all the grays. I wish I had an A+ in handling the pain, too.

THE NEXT LAP

After the immense pain, I went to my urologist to find a solution and to remove the catheter from my bladder. While we were in the exam room, he got a call from the hospital from a certain Dr. Rao, who was a pathologist with the same surname as mine. There was some confusion, and he left the room as the calling pathologist had informed it to be urgent. He came back looking grim and dropped the bombshell. The pathologist was calling with my report, and it was urgent because he found malignant cells in my lesion and seeing a 30-year-old woman with bladder cancer cells was urgent indeed. Until today, I don't know how Suresh and I made it back home. Both of us were crying and I am baffled how Suresh was able to see the road with tears brimming in his eyes.

The severity of the diagnosis had not fully set in. I was thankful that the cancer was in my native kidney and not in my transplanted one. My solace was that surgically removing the kidney should not affect the quality of life. My urologist offered to perform the surgery within ten days. There was still this tiny matter of what to tell the family. Should we just say it was a cyst and a benign surgical removal to make it easier for my family, or should we divulge the diagnosis?

We decided to go with the former with only my sisters knowing the true story. As luck would have it, Suresh's uncle and aunt had already planned to visit us during the time of surgery and were with us for ten days during that difficult time. Having them around helped elevate the mood as they were a friendly couple. Of course, they were dutifully informed that it was a surgery to remove some type of cyst in my kidney.

On December 14, 2004, I underwent a long surgery to remove my native right kidney, along with the ureter all the way to the bladder cuff. This surgery was a feather in my surgeon's hat, as he had to do a lot of maneuvering to reach my kidney. Betsy, as my transplanted kidney was fondly called, was sitting on top of the ureter of my right kidney and so he could not reach the bladder cuff. Betsy and I were harmonious, I was happy with her location in my body, and she was cozily settled in. To ensure Betsy was not harmed, he devised an innovative method of going into my bladder and reaching the ureter junction from the inside. Surgery continued until very late in the evening, and I was transferred to the recovery ward somewhere during the night.

SMALL BLESSINGS

We were given a taste of the dismissive side of the American medical system after three days when my doctor decided to discharge me with at least three tubes hanging out and my pain still fairly high. We were not prepared for my homecoming at all, other than moving the bed downstairs. This was an incision surgery where my lowest right rib was removed and the largest muscle on the right side of my waist was cut through, to reach the kidney. Saying I was in immense pain in every single position would be an understatement. A urinary catheter was not helping either.

We were totally not prepared for the tornado that hit us that night. The only preparation we had done for my homecoming was moving the bed from upstairs to downstairs. We had the foresight that with pain and catheters, it would be tough for one to climb the stairs. How many engineers does it take to plan for a surgery homecoming? Two naïve junior engineers.

The first night was filled with fitful sleep dosed with Tylenol. We decided to bring in the forces the next day, and our dear friend Srikrishnan was the man of the hour. Srikrishnan is a very close childhood friend of Suresh and an equally close friend of mine from our college days. He is that friend who cares for you during all hardships and with you every step of the way. He is more of a family member of our household; his family is an extension of our family. We are very lucky to have a friend like Srikrishnan with us for the past umpteen years.

Ten days after surgery, my dear, always loving mother landed in California to take care of me. We decided to let my mother know that it was cancer and not some simple cyst. She was naïve concerning cancer and needed some reassurance that it would be all fine. After ten days, thankfully, my catheter and other tubes came out. I was walking inside the house holding on to my urine bag by then and was raring to gain my freedom from the catheter. Why me? Why me? The question that haunts every single cancer patient. I had no answer for why. Why indeed! If we all had clear explanations for the happenings in this universe, life would be simple. The human body remains a mystery to us all.

On December 26, twelve days after my surgery, I was watching TV when the news of a devastating tsunami hitting most coastal cities in India, resulting in a lot of deaths, reached us. Compared to those suffering in India in the aftermath of the tsunami, I felt lucky at that moment for having detected cancer early, having it removed, and sipping hot chocolate in the comfort of my home. It was more of why not me, instead of why me?

7 Chemotherapy
Look For The Ray Of Sunshine

"I THINK CHEMOTHERAPY is the treatment where people lose their hair," I said.

"Are you sure? I don't think you will need that treatment. Your tumor has already been removed," said Suresh.

UROLOGIST, ONCOLOGIST AND URO-ONCOLOGIST

That was our conversation outside the urologist's office when I went for a follow up after the surgery. We were naïve and had no clue about the treatment for cancer. In my naivety, I assumed getting rid of the tumor by surgery would cure me of the disease. I had no understanding about the grades or stages of cancer. The only stage I was familiar with was Shakespeare's world stage where we were all supposed to be players.

The pathology report came back, validating that the cancer was stage 3, which is a very advanced stage of cancer. That was enough to send a shiver up my spine, especially when I was unaware of what that even meant. My urologist, Dr. Aigen, referred me to an oncologist, Dr Wu in the same clinic. While sitting at the oncologist's office, neither Suresh nor I had any clue what to expect. I was more worried about losing my hair than all the other side effects of chemotherapy. Little did I know how wrong I was then.

To my pleasant surprise, Dr. Wu was the most genuine and friendly doctor I had ever met. As soon as she read my case history, she was honest enough to admit that she would want me to consult with a senior doctor, specializing in urological oncology, at Stanford Hospital. She did not want to make any decision on her own without a second opinion.

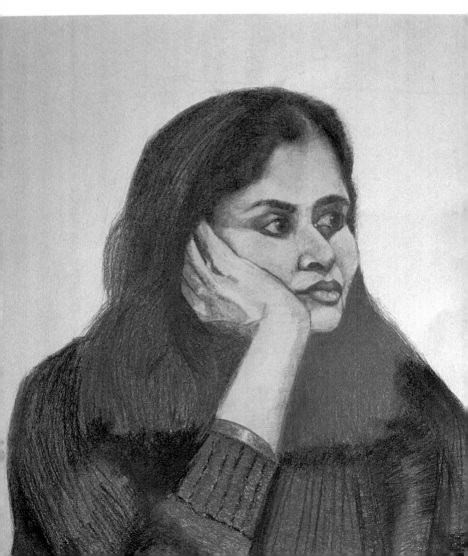

When I first met Dr. Sandy at Stanford Hospital, I was incredibly impressed by the clarity with which she explained all the details of the disease, the treatment, and the statistics. It was comforting to see a radiologist, a urologist, and a urologic oncologist in the same room, all discussing the treatment options with me. I was informed that I will be having chemo treatment to get rid of any microscopic cells that could have been missed, followed by radiation therapy if needed.

I applied for a leave of absence at work and decided to go on short-term disability. Luckily, my work insurance was excellent and comprehensive. I was covered for every penny that was needed for the therapy.

MOP-UP CHEMO

Chemotherapy is portrayed with a picture of patients with bald heads so much that we have come to symbolize cancer with bald heads. It is the ubiquitous mark of a suffering cancer patient. Chemo treatments are a lot more than just losing hair. The amount of side effects varies from patient to patient depending on the drug used as well as the patient's genetic makeup. It affects your body and brain, taxing you physically, emotionally, and mentally. It is equivalent to climbing a snowy mountain with no shoes on, your body shivering, being out of breath due to the lack of oxygen and your brain screaming at the Almighty to stop the brutality. You wish for it to be a nightmare from which you can come out eventually only to be sucked back in at the beginning of every cycle of the treatment.

I was prescribed three cycles of mop-up chemotherapy. It is fondly called mop-up because it is trying to mop up all the left-over malignant cells. I never knew I would hate and love mopping at the same time. All my tumors had been removed by the surgery. I was essentially boasting what we call an NED (no evidence of disease) in the cancer world. NED reflects the absence of visible cells while scanning the body. But this scan doesn't guarantee the absence of lurking cancer cells which are not visible, which could be blissfully mutating, growing, and thriving.

If Darwin were alive today, he would be ecstatic to note the fighting spirit of the cancer cells. The human race has not been able to beat them for centuries. To evade these masters in sleight, I had to undergo four cycles of chemo treatment. My therapy drug was a combination of cisplatin and gemcitabine, typically called "Gemzar" (its brand name) by doctors and patients.

Unfortunately, as luck would have it, the drug cisplatin used for bladder cancer is highly toxic to the kidneys. I was not happy about it, and neither was Betsy, the nickname I had given to my transplanted kidney. Seriously, imagine being Betsy for a moment. She had to do all her regular chores alone which other kidneys do along with a mate, only to be bombarded with chemicals as a reward. My oncologist had a plan how not to put too much stress on Betsy's functions. She planned to admit me to the hospital for a couple of days, administer the chemo drug, and start hydrating me immediately to flush the toxins out of the kidney. She did mention that this might affect my fertility. Suresh and I were planning on kids, but we put everything on hold due to the cancer. Later, we did decide not to have any children.

My chemo regimen was the first week cisplatin plus gemzar, the second week gemzar, then off chemo the third week. Since the therapy doesn't hit you immediately, I was working the first week of my treatment, with plans to take a leave of absence the following week. A common side effect of chemo is nausea, which is well studied and controlled by drugs, assuming one takes them without fail. With my transplant, I was already used to taking medications every single day. Adding one more drug did not affect me, and I was very diligent.

But, a few days into the treatment, when I was at work saying my goodbyes to colleagues, I almost fainted due to a high fever. That morning, I woke up with a slightly elevated temperature which I ignored and merrily went on my way to work to say my goodbyes. I came home by lunch time and crashed on the couch, burning hot. I went to my room to lie down and asked my mother not to disturb me even for lunch.

BLOOD TEST RESULTS

Luckily, I had taken a blood test just the day before and I got a call from the doc's office when Suresh and mom were wondering what to do. Apparently, I had neutropenic fever, which you get due to neutropenia, loss of WBC (white blood cells) in your blood. The normal count of WBC in our blood is around 4K to 10K for an adult and my count was at 1K. I was asked to immediately rush to the clinic to get neupogen shots, which helped in boosting the WBC. The standard dose is to get the shot for five days. After five days, I was feeling a lot better with no fever but with a lot of body pain.

When checked again, my WBC was at 100K. Ten times the normal count. This is what happens when drug dosage standards are based on a thirty-year-old, 5' 10' Caucasian male weighing 155 pounds. No wonder that a petite, 5' 1", 100-pound Asian woman like me was over dosed. Every single drug dosage for most ailments is determined after trials on men, except for certain drugs for pregnancy and other ailments that affect only women.

I hope the future generation bring the change we need with a lot more inclusivity for women. When we design everything from cars, to air-conditioned offices, to city streets, we reference men as the default user. And when it comes to healthcare, that can mean deadly effects for women.

Neupogen is a bone marrow stimulant which is notorious for causing severe bone pain throughout the body. This pain affected me even more than the chemotherapy side effects. When one's body is in pain, the scream stops at the throat and doesn't come out. There is no energy for the scream to escape. Soaking in a hot tub just makes you damp with no solace for the pain. The icing on this painful cake was getting five shots that unnecessarily increased my pain. Having learned the lesson, my dosage was reduced to one shot for the rest of my cycles.

As mentioned, cisplatin, belonging to the platinum family of chemo drugs, has an adverse effect on the kidneys. Common side effects include bone marrow suppression, hearing problems sometimes leading to hearing loss, vomiting and kidney function issues. It has been used since the 1990s for cancer treatment. After a couple cycles into the treatment, my creatinine levels started rising indicating a doomsday scenario for poor Betsy, my petite transplanted kidney. I was secretly feeling thrilled as this might mean a stop to the chemo treatment. As badly as I wanted to get cured of the cancer, that immediate reprieve from chemo loomed big, making me forget about everything else.

It was very tough handling the side effects of cisplatin. My ears were buzzing all the time. I could not stand even a slight increase in volume, be it the television or someone talking loudly. From the age of twenty-five, after my transplant, I suffered from tinnitus with a constant whooshing sound in my ears. Now, with cisplatin, there was mayhem inside my ears. There was a constant cacophony going on in my head. I supposed at the time that all the sounds were battling to figure out who could finally make me deaf.

Finally, the battle in my ears came to an end with the decision to take me off cisplatin due to its damaging effect on my kidney. My creatinine was at 1.5 milligrams per deciliter, a tad bit over what is deemed normal. It reached 1.5 after just two cycles with the initial value at the start being 0.9. These levels are not really a scenario one would want to have develop.

NEW DRUG REGIMEN

My oncologists decided to switch me to a different regimen, carboplatin with gemcitabine. Carboplatin is another drug from the same platinum family as cisplatin, used for treating various types of cancers. It is essentially a cousin of cisplatin. Since it was supposed to be less lethal to the kidneys, I did not have to get admitted to the hospital while the drugs were being administered. The side effects of carboplatin were milder but instead of WBC, my red blood cells dipped too low. In layman's terms, I was becoming anemic.

Not a surprise, as no chemo is a breeze. A rose bush is always filled with thorns, however beautiful it might look. You must get pricked, literally and figuratively to survive a chemo regimen. I got pricked every week with a needle, either for delivering chemo or receiving blood to counter the side effects or just to get my blood tested. For someone with ultra-thin and deep veins, this was always a nightmare. *Sometimes, one must suffer through the nightmares in their sleep, to wake up to life.*

FAMILY AND FRIENDS

There I was, in the middle of the nightmare, always waiting eagerly to wake up. There is always something to look forward to in life, amid all the hurdles. With Suresh and my mother both being by my side, it was made rosy enough, with more roses than thorns when I woke up from my nightmare. To make me feel better, my friends Padma and Susheela visited me during my chemo ordeal to help me keep going.

A waft of friendly air amid suffering can cheer anyone up. By the time my second cycle was done, I was completely bald with a few strands of hair only at the back. With those strands of hair jutting out of my head, it was quite comical, and I tried to evoke a laugh or two from others by trying to show that hair off. Laughter is the best medicine after all. To find humor during suffering has always helped me plow through it. *Life is a journey that is best taken in a vehicle loaded with humor and laughter.*

During the whole time, there was another ray of sunshine who visited me every other week. It was my friends Srikrishnan and Saumya's daughter, Keena. She was born just around the time I was diagnosed. A bubbly, ever smiling, pretty little doll, she was a very happy child who made everything around her rosier. Today, even as a teenager, she is a ray of sunshine whenever she visits us. After my chemotherapy ended, I visited my friends every weekend just to have some quality time with this little darling. A moment of pure happiness and bliss amid anguish. A perfect godchild who any godmother could have wished for.

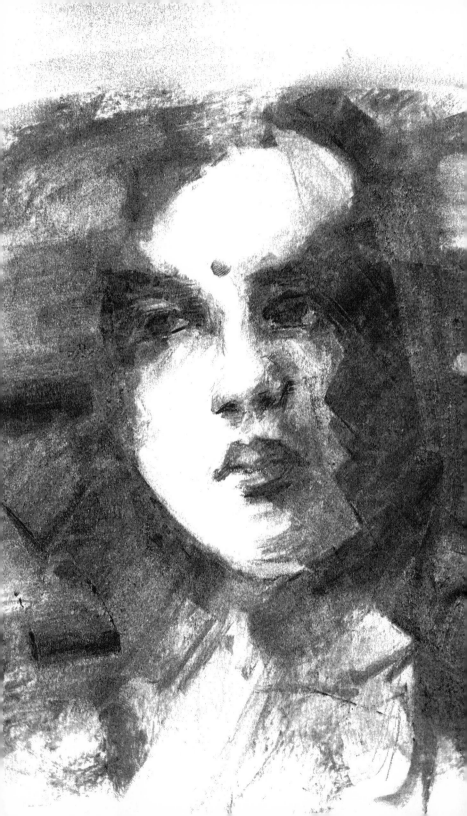

8 Lifestyle
Your Body Is Your Temple

"WHY IS CANCER A TABOO?" I lamented to Suresh.

When I was first diagnosed with cancer, we could not share it with many, other than a few close friends. There were a couple of good reasons. We did not want to worry our parents and we thought there was no point in telling people unless the topic came up. But, hiding it from others was very tough.

CANCER IS TABOO

My mother was the only parent who knew as she was taking care of me. We kept the news from dad as he was alone in India while mom was with me in California. We determined that informing Suresh's parents was not a good idea because we were not sure what the reaction or repercussions would be. I personally was afraid to let them know as I was already ridden with guilt from holding back Suresh in life due to my numerous health hurdles. I was quite confident that this might make them angry at me for spoiling their son's life, which would have been a natural response for an Asian parent in those days. I was afraid that I might hold back Suresh professionally due to my needs. I made a resolution that day not to ever let my health hurdles come in the way of our life, especially Suresh's.

But then, every week when we called home to India, we had to act normal despite abnormal and painful events at home. Thankfully, there were no free apps then for video calls so most of our calls to my dad and in-laws were only voice calls over the phone. Reflecting on that episode of my life, I wonder if we could have acted differently by involving others, especially parents who as our well-wishers might have made them feel included and made our pain less painful.

Keeping it private from parents might not have been a good idea but from others definitely so. When I went back to work, it seemed that everyone had a cancer story of how an uncle died, how an aunt fully recovered from breast cancer, or how they can understand my situation just because one of their friend's roommates had cancer.

Often, when people hear of someone who has battled cancer or is going through treatments, they reply with the statement, "Sorry. Be strong." Some take it to the next level and discuss how their cousin once removed suffered from skin cancer thus inherently somehow making them experts on all types of cancers. I learned one important lesson in all my discussions with people who have not been touched by this disease. They can be sympathetic but not empathetic unless they have seen hardships in life. When encountering folks who have not seen hurdles in life, I have decided to keep quiet and not share my cancer journey. If shared, it often is awkward for them and me, resulting in unnecessary heartbreak and stress.

I was very happy with those who barely mentioned it and accepted me as I was. A shaved head with new growing hair was giving enough clues for some despite my silence. I wore a wig initially, waiting for a tiny bit of hair to show up on my head before removing the wig. That day arrived within a couple of weeks. On removing the wig and exposing my head, I felt liberated as though I had renewed myself.

RENEWAL

Indeed, I was a new person both inside and out. I had morphed to be more empathetic emotionally while physically, I had lost a lot of weight. Indeed, I felt like a renewed person with a burst of energy, able to enjoy my freedom. I rocked my new look with a lot of confidence, so much so that I received compliments from people who were unaware of my chemo treatments. A summer hair-cut, I would proclaim loudly and proudly.

Cancer awakens you to the journey of living that you barely registered before and scraped through. I became very conscious of what went into my body. My diet included organic vegetables, fruits, nuts, and whole grains. Breakfast was oatmeal with blueberries or milk with fruits. Living close to work had its perks and I was able to have a healthy lunch with homemade salad and fresh Indian food loaded with vegetables. Every afternoon, I drove home to have a fresh, hot lunch. Looking after my diet and changing my lifestyle took precedence in life. After my kidney transplant, I was very careful about not eating anything raw due to my suppressed immunity, but now I searched for restaurants that would serve healthy food. The days of binging on donuts were over.

While researchers continue to investigate the connection between sugar and cancer, there is accumulating evidence that sugar consumption is associated with increased cancer risk, recurrence, and mortality. Specifically, high blood sugar levels lead to conditions such as high insulin levels and obesity, which both increase the risk for cancer.

LIFESTYLE AND NUTRITION

As much as the doctors say there is no correlation between sugar and cancer, I refuse to believe it to this day. Knowing sugar is bad not just for cancer but for myriad other reasons, initially, I stopped eating sugar in any form. The further I moved away from my therapies, I did indulge every now and then. My lunch often had salad as one of the dishes along with some healthy grains. Quinoa and whole wheat were the norm though my Indian gene that craved for rice had to be satisfied frequently. Being a vegetarian from birth, it was easy to avoid meat and animal protein. Being an Indian, adding turmeric, ginger, garlic to our food was a given and one that I diligently followed in every meal. Indian cuisine with its use of all kinds of spices and condiments was the norm in our household and that made eating healthy very easy.

I was new to baking but the zest for healthy eating made me master the art. As often said, baking is a science and my engineering brain had to devise various ways of making my baked goodies healthy. It was a challenge but one that I enjoyed in myriad ways. I understood the basics of all the necessary ingredients and how they react with each other so I could use the right substitutes for unhealthy ingredients. Sugar was substituted with dates and bananas. All-purpose flour was often substituted with a mix of oat flour and whole wheat flour. Apple sauce for oil or butter. Purists would argue that it may not be tasty, but if I can eat a chocolate cake that is healthy and tastes like chocolate, I would take it. It was a pleasure to share my goodies with my friends.

What is the use of healthy food if you don't move your arms and legs to work with the healthy part? And so started the exercises at the gym, dance workouts, and walking regularly. I was introduced to meditation by one of my friends and that has helped me to this day.

BONDING WITH TRAVEL

From 2005 to 2011, life was bliss, filled with fun, excitement, and lots of travel. Life was normal, albeit a new normal, with ongoing scans. But our lives were switched on at full speed, and Suresh and I enjoyed every ounce of it. Initially, after the chemo, I had to undergo MRI scans every three months for three years, followed by scans every six months for two more years, finally progressing to yearly scans. The scans are done to look for any cancer recurrence in my body. For bladder cancers, the doctors also do a procedure called cystoscopy, which is essentially scoping your bladder to look for abnormalities.

Every scan was a nightmare to endure with an anxious mind fearing the worst most often. We planned our travel around the scans. We never made any plans that went beyond six months. It was as exciting as it was surprising since we decided at the last minute. We visited the UK, France, Greece, Germany, Italy, New Zealand, and many more countries other than our usual visits to India.

For a couple without children, there were no major school commitments, so we were good to go if we could make time in our work schedule. My work took me to places, too, especially countries in Asia. Visiting countries with different cultures and languages is always a pleasure because one's knowledge about the world grows. To this day, I enjoy planning for our trips. I meticulously go through all the important sightseeing that needs to be done, places to visit, how to make it fun and unique, all the right hotels to stay in, and restaurants to cater to our foodie stomachs.

GIVING BACK

As soon as I recovered from chemo, by the end of 2005, I started volunteering with the Cancer Institute Foundation (CIF). CIF is a non-profit organization that helps with raising funds for the Adyar Cancer Institute in Chennai, India. It is an institute and hospital that caters to very poor patients by giving them free cancer care. Every dollar matters, since it is a purely volunteer-driven organization, there is no overhead. I volunteered at CIF helping with their fundraising efforts, most often by organizing various events. As karma would have it, I met Dr. Sandy from Stanford University personally while organizing events, as she was one of the doctors who passionately helped CIF in various ways. She is the same uro-oncologist who had advised me for my chemotherapy treatment.

9 Bladder Cancer
Listen To Your Instincts

"WHY DID YOU book the cystoscopy appointment on January 3?" cried Suresh. "I have an important meeting and am busy the whole day."

CONSISTENCY

Once an appointment is obtained, you don't skip it. That was my mantra. Hence, we were at the urologist's office promptly at 2 p.m. for the cystoscopy appointment. After my recovery from chemo, I had to have my bladder scoped frequently, to check for cancer. My cancer was diagnosed in my ureter which has a lining of bladder cells, henceforth, the possibility of it recurring in the bladder was very high.

The plan was to get scoped every three months for three years, every six months for two years after, and finally once a year for ten years. It had been seven years since my diagnosis of cancer in the ureter of my native kidney, when I went in for scoping that day. Dr. Aigen, my urologist, walked in with a smile greeting us as usual and peeked into my bladder with the scope. Regardless of the number of cystoscopies I have done, I am always nervous during the appointment.

Though it was like any other regular cystoscopy appointment, my gut was telling me that something was not right that day. My gut feeling told me there might be a problem, though it was seven years out from my first diagnosis of cancer.

Within a minute of peeking into the bladder, Dr. Aigen said, "I see a new tumor".

"What?" I cried.

As much as I had felt the harbinger of doom that morning, I was not ready to hear it. I started crying immediately. It felt like the tears were waiting to flow out that morning and found a release. My instincts are never wrong.

Suresh and I both were stumped and lost our bearings. It took a while to come to our senses and extreme willpower to walk out of the exam room, through the hospital corridors, and finally making it to our cars. Since it was a weekday, we both had taken our cars and had driven to the clinic from work. Thinking about what happened that day, I am relieved and amazed that we decided to go back to work.

BACK TO WORK

Yes, go back to work. I was back at my desk in thirty minutes, looking at a budget approval. My boss noticed something was wrong and called me over to talk. With tears brimming in my eyes, I told him that my cancer had returned.

I don't know how I managed to work the entire day. That evening, I went home, not sure how to feel about it. I informed our close friends who have been like family in the US; they came running to console me and provide their support. My friend Srikrishnan and his wife

Saumya are the best friends anyone could hope for; I am so grateful that they came right over to our home even though it was late at night when they heard the news.

My other friend, Hema, who is my sister from another mother, was equally shattered. An empathetic human, she views me as her younger sister and is super protective when it comes to my well-being. The very next day after the diagnosis, she invited Suresh and I for dinner, helped me cry out my anxiety, and provided a shoulder to cry upon. Until today, she is one of the few people in my life to whom I run when I need assurance, protection, discussion, and just listening. I am eternally grateful to all these friends.

THE NEXT LAP OF MY RACE

Once the initial shock of the diagnosis was past, my brain started analyzing the situation like an engineer. As an engineer, I always looked at every single situation as a problem waiting for a solution. I decided to be calm until after my TURB (transurethral resection of the bladder) that will tell us how big and how far into the muscle the tumor has invaded. Dr. Aigen scheduled a TURB within a few days and I proceeded with the surgery.

During the TURB, my tumor was removed for further biopsy and analysis. It was an outpatient surgery with only Suresh accompanying me to the clinic, waiting patiently outside while the surgery was ongoing. I was in the recovery room for a couple of hours before leaving for home with a catheter dangling out of my bladder. I walked out holding on to the catheter with my head held high, albeit in pain.

I was never ashamed of catheters. After my surgery for upper tract TCC (transitional cell cancer) seven years back, I had to wear the catheter for ten days before it was removed. I remember proudly walking into the small clinic, holding my bag of pee in one hand, the bag dangling from under my skirt. There were some awkward stares and smiles from other patients. But, hey, it was a urologist's office after all.

NON-METASTATIC BLADDER CANCER

After my TURB, I took full bed rest for a couple of days with Suresh taking care of my dietary needs. Saumya, who I call the Energizer Bunny, took off from work and visited us in the mornings to help Suresh out. The pathology report came back within a couple of days indicating that I had high grade bladder cancer which had not invaded the muscle. It was superficial, the best news one could hope for when talking about bladder cancer. It was stage 0. Cancer is the only disease where the lower number gets the better prognosis. That gave us both immense relief.

The disease looked like a beast that could be beatable. My heart said I could handle it. The other reason for the relief was the fact that I didn't have to do another surgery. A few days back, Dr. Aigen had suggested that he might want to cut into my bladder again just to ensure that there was no muscle involvement as he was not sure how deep he cut while removing the tumor. But when the pathology showed margins saying the tumor had not penetrated even the topmost epithelial layer, he deemed it unnecessary. Just when I was about to let out a sigh of relief, Dr. Aigen said that it might be a good idea to remove the bladder and build a new one with my intestines.

PERSPECTIVE MATTERS

For people with advanced but non-metastatic bladder cancer, removing the bladder is normal. Taking my age into account, my urologist wanted to be very aggressive and remove the bladder. I was rattled enough as it was and was not ready to give up my bladder. One important lesson I have learned over the years is that every doctor looks at a problem from their perspective to come up with a solution. From a urologist's perspective, the best aggressive treatment was the removal of the bladder.

The bladder tumor was at the cuff of the bladder, the place where the ureter attached to my native left kidney, meets the bladder. Though I heaved a sigh of relief on finding that my bladder cancer was superficial and categorized as stage 0, I still had my doubts about going for a bladder removal.

I turned to Dr. Sandy from Stanford Hospital, who specialized in urology. Due to my volunteer work helping the Cancer Institute Foundation, I had come to know Dr. Sandy well enough that I could call her in my time of distress. She immediately referred me to Dr. Gill at Stanford, a well-known urologist, to get a second opinion. Stanford Center also did a pathology of my tumor, which came back as stage 0. Dr. Gill advised me to do mitomycin chemo treatments to the bladder, same as my urologist. Of course, the well-known caveat was added to the answer, "It might work—no one can guarantee."

In general, for bladder cancer, the prescribed treatment is the administration of intravesical BCG (expansion). BCG is a bacterium that causes tuberculosis. A low dose of BCG is put into the bladder which increases the body's immunity to fight against anything attacking the bladder. For someone who is already immunosuppressed and relies on the same for survival, BCG did not seem like a good idea. Hence, mitomycin came into the picture. It was also the prescribed treatment for those who could not afford to get BCG.

The prescribed course was intravesical mitomycin to be delivered into my bladder every week for three months, then, every month for six months. Intravesical means delivering the medicine straight into the bladder through a catheter tube. Thus, the second chemo course of my life started. Every visit was an adventure. The nurses had a tough time finding my urethra every single time. Most often, the first insertion was in my vagina. I had this constant fear that one day they might deliver mitomycin into my ureter instead of the bladder. It was too close for comfort. The nurses generally found it at the second try, so I must give credit where it is due. Luckily, evolution did not consider it necessary for another hole in the same vicinity, which would have added to my anxiety.

I was asked to roll around for a couple of hours after the injection of mitomycin to ensure it spread all over the bladder. I started rolling as soon as I reached home. If we had a dog then, it would have enjoyed rolling with me for sure. That is exactly what I was doing, belly up and rolling from side to side every few minutes. What fun! I would have never thought my life would involve rolling around like a dog one day. Life indeed takes you through weird turns and twists.

TOASTMASTERS

While rolling around on the bed, I was rolling on with public speaking as well. In 2011, I had joined a Toastmasters club near my house. Every Saturday morning at 8:00a.m., I was fresh and ready to network with a set of people from diverse backgrounds to enhance my public speaking skills. From childhood, I was a consistent contestant in my school's elocution contests. Though it was most often written by my sister Hema, I was good at memorizing and delivering the speeches. I was always the most expressive kid around the block. On joining Toastmasters, to my pleasant surprise, I found that I was good at not just delivering speeches but writing them, too. To hone the skills further and just to meet others with the same interests, my toastmasters journey continues until this day. Over the years, I served in various leadership positions as well which helped me learn more about service leadership rather than an authoritarian one.

Bladder cancer did not stop me from continuing my speeches. I remember vividly how surprised my friend was one day when she learned that I had postponed my intravesical mitomycin insertion just so I could be a Toastmaster for one of the area contests. If mitomycin and public speaking cannot travel together, wonder how life would have been?

10 Why Not Me?

Research Your Disease

"FINALLY! YEA! Last day of treatment", I shouted.

"Let us celebrate", Suresh chimed in, and we treated ourselves to a nice spa treatment and dinner.

As much as I was elated to be finished with the treatments, there was always the nagging question "Why me?" When I was diagnosed with bladder cancer the second time, my brain was screaming "Why me?" I had followed all the right protocols and suggestions. I cut down on sugar, eating only nutritious, organic food with less grains, more vegetables, fruits, and fiber-rich foods.

I was also regularly exercising with Suresh's support. In the interval of seven years from my first cancer, Suresh had started running marathons and relays. From a 185-pound young man with a paunch, he had transformed into a muscular, very fit man because of running. This had motivated me to start jogging, strength training with regular walking on the side. I don't want you to assume that I became a fitness freak. It was just something I tried to keep myself fit. I was very surprised when I was diagnosed with bladder cancer despite being fit and eating healthy.

The question "Why me?" played on a loop in my head. As someone who is analytical and thinks like an engineer, always looking for a logical explanation for everything that life throws at me, I started researching. With so many years behind the invention of the internet, data was at all our fingertips, literally and figuratively.

RESEARCH HELPS YOU BE YOUR OWN ADVOCATE

During my research, I read various articles on bladder cancer and kidney failure. There were hundreds of posts on bladder cancer, with the causes always pointing to smoking, hair dye and a few other chemicals. I was confident I had never smoked in my life with no passive smoking exposure either. If the one time I dyed my hair brown could be taken as exposure, then that was the only explanation I could think of. Maybe, in that one dyeing, I got close to dying.

While going through various bladder cancer articles, I hit upon one paper submitted by a few doctors in a Belgium study. A group of women in Belgium had opted to take a Chinese herbal medicine as part of their weight-loss regimen.[2]

Unfortunately, the herbs got mixed up and instead of the weight loss herb, their medicine had *aristolochia indica* in it. Apparently, this herb was toxic to the kidneys if taken for a long duration. This herb can cause a gene mutation in your DNA, in this case, the DNA found in the kidney and urinary tract. Most of the women, depending on their dosage, ended up with kidney failure. The paper went on further to describe how these women tended to get cancer in the ureter, due to which the doctors generally removed the native kidneys while transplanting a new one. If this coincidence was not enough, guess what? Despite the removal of the native kidneys, most patients developed a bladder tumor a few years after the transplant. The prognosis of the bladder cancer varied depending on when it was discovered, though most did not go past stage 2.

NATURAL IS NOT EQUIVALENT TO SAFE

Reading the paper gave me chills and I was pretty sure that this was not a coincidence. The only treatment that I had ever had in my life before the failure, was the herbal medicine for my vitiligo. Herbal medicines, belonging to the specific alternative medicine called 'Siddha', practiced mostly in South India, were medicines of trust and loyalty. You never asked the doctor what herbs went into them even if you were well-educated, let alone the child that I was.

I did not let this fact hinder me; I scoured the internet about the treatments for vitiligo in Siddha medicine. Sure enough, after a couple of tries, I hit upon an article showing all the concoctions used for vitiligo.[3] There was the culprit. The villain in my story. For treating vitiligo, three herb mixtures were used, one of which was '*aristolochia indica*', known as Indian birthwort, which was nephrotoxic.

This plant contains aristolochic acid, a carcinogen also found in various *aristolochia* and *asarum* plants, both in the family *aristolochiaceae*. Aristolochic acid is composed of about 1:1 mixture of two forms, aristolochic acid I and aristolochic acid II.

In addition to its carcinogenicity, aristolochic acid is also highly nephrotoxic, which in layman's terms means toxic to the kidneys. In fact, it is known to be a causative agent for what is termed as Balkan nephropathy.

Balkan endemic nephropathy (BEN) is a form of interstitial nephritis, which is an inflammation of the kidneys that causes kidney failure. First identified in the 1920s among several small communities along the Danube River and its major tributaries, it is caused by small long-term doses of aristolochic acid in the diet. BEN Is also found in the modern countries of Croatia, Bosnia and Herzegovina, Serbia, Romania, and Bulgaria.

The disease primarily affects people thirty to sixty years of age. Doses of the toxin are usually low and people moving to endemic areas typically develop the condition only when they have lived there for ten to twenty years. People taking higher doses of aristolochic acid (as Chinese herbal supplements) have developed kidney failure after shorter durations of exposure. These patients are distinguished from those suffering from other causes of end-stage renal disease by showing an absence of high blood pressure, xanthochromia of palms and soles (Tanchev's sign), early hypochromic anemia, absence of proteinuria, and slow progression of kidney failure.[4]

This explained why I did not have high blood pressure and dominant anemia as well as my progression to failure being slow unlike some of the other reasons for kidney failure. Patients with this type of failure have a greatly increased rate of transitional cell carcinoma (TCC) of the upper urothelial tract, (the renal pelvis and ureters) after a few years , which explained why I got cancer in my ureter seven years after my kidney transplant.

The explanation of my kidney failure did not stop there. Aristolochic acid preferentially binds to purines in the DNA and is associated with a high frequency of A-->T transversions in the p53 gene. The *TP53* gene provides instructions for making a protein called tumor protein p53 (or p53). This protein acts as a tumor suppressor, which means that it regulates cell division by keeping cells from growing and dividing (proliferating) too fast or in an uncontrolled way. Anyone with mutations in this gene are prone to cancer, as once triggered the cells divide uncontrollably, that is the description of cancer growth.[5]

So finally, there was the answer to the question "Why me?" Now I know why. My symptoms followed all the classic cases of poisoning by that herb. Kidney failure, followed by transplant, upper tract ureter cancer and seven years later, bladder cancer. This cause and effect could not have been clearer.

I had a mixed feeling of relief and loss interspersed with a lot of what-ifs. Relief that there was logic behind the suffering. It was not like one day God decided to say, 'And so, you shall suffer'. My feeling of loss was mainly due to all the missed events in life due to this disease. What if I hadn't gotten vitiligo? What if I had not taken herbal medicine? What if I had removed both my kidneys while having the transplant? There were thousands of what-ifs running in my brain, but the relief overtook everything after a few days, bringing in a much needed feeling of calm. I knew the enemy now and was ready to fight.

I resolved to do whatever it takes to fight this disease

and live life to the fullest, with whatever had been handed out to me. With this knowledge came the realization that I still had one of my native kidneys, intact in my body. I showed the papers to my urologist, explaining about the herb and the sequence of events. He immediately understood the significance of the removal of the remaining kidney.

My bladder tumor had occurred very close to the cuff, where the left ureter meets the bladder. As much as I was afraid of cancer cells spreading outside the bladder during the surgery, I was determined to take the risk.

KIDNEY REMOVAL

In February 2012, I was wheeled in for one more surgery, a robotic surgery this time. This was the first robotic surgery for my urologist, but I was ready to be his first patient. Anything for science and technological advancement. Recovery from the surgery was very fast, much to our relief. The scars were minimal with no muscle involvement, unlike the surgery I had seven years back to remove my other kidney.

Technology and advancement in science has saved me time and again, along with good doctors. I had the catheter in for ten days and the recuperation was fast once it came out. Unlike the previous time, we were prepared and determined not to get discharged too early from the hospital. In my previous stint, discharge after three days led to extreme suffering at home. After this surgery, I ensured that all tubes and paraphernalia came out except for the catheter before getting discharged.

There is a huge difference in how medical care works in India and the United States. During my kidney transplant, my mother and I were hospitalized a day in advance, just so we didn't get too nervous while the prep for surgery was ongoing. After the transplant, both of us stayed in the hospital for one full week while recuperating. Using the Indian medical system requires a mix of insurance coverage and self-pay. I suppose this plays a major factor. When I had my kidney removal surgery in 2004, I was hospitalized the day of the surgery, and asked to leave the hospital within three days. We found it very difficult to manage it at home. You are a burden for the insurance company if they are paying for you. This was a major surgery where I went back home with three tubes hanging out at various locations. I am pretty sure if it were India, the doctors would not have discharged me unless they were sure of my medical status.

With both my native kidneys removed and the intravesical chemo helping my bladder further, I felt as though life was on the mend. A new normal yet again. My mother, the caretaking diva that she was, spent a couple of months helping me sort out my feelings after the surgery and recovery. Nothing works like a charm better than a mother's cooking. For all my other needs, I had my 24/7 caretaker, my husband Suresh. Of all the what-ifs of my life, I always wonder "What if I had not met Suresh and fallen in love?" I cannot fathom a life without him. He is my superhero.

11 Angiosarcoma
Be Your Own Advocate

"MS. RAO, WE WOULD like you to get the CD of your scan. The report says there is a lesion in your liver," said the nurse during the call.

My mind reeled and feared the worst. Could it be because of too many activities? It had been few months since I had started an LLC, Scoop and Bake, along with my friend Hema. Wanting to be entrepreneurs, coupled with our passion for baking, a cookie business had seemed just right. Along with our day work, creating an LLC, website, and working on weekends for the same seemed fine. "But I was not stressed at all", screamed my brain.

JUMPING THE NEXT HURDLE
The year was 2014. It was just two years after my latest kidney removal surgery. I was at work when the call came. I had taken my follow-up MRI scan a couple of days back and was waiting nervously for the results. In the cancer world, we call it "scanxiety." As it so often happens, you get an important call least when you expect it. The call came when I was walking along the corridor after an important meeting, totally immersed in work. It took me a few minutes to understand what she was asking. Lesion? In my liver? The bladder is fine? CD of my MRI scan? The same questions were rotating in my head for quite a while. Before the news reached my brain, my

stomach started churning with fear, the queasy feeling of fear which overshadows all emotions within you.

Whenever I face fear, I remember the quote from Frank Herbert's, *Dune*[6]:

> *"I must not fear.*
> *Fear is the mind-killer.*
> *Fear is the little death that brings total obliteration.*
> *I will face my fear."*

Regardless of how many times you might have heard the statement, "We found something. It could be cancer," it hits you anew every single time. There is no "been there, done that" when it comes to cancer. The fear sets in without fail. Then the tears make their presence known, followed by panic.

LIVER LESION

I walked back to my desk, eyes brimming with tears and called Suresh immediately. It felt like the world was collapsing around me, taking Suresh along with me. It had been only a couple of years since my bladder cancer. Already another one? What could the liver lesion be?

As an engineer my immediate response was to search the internet for all possible causes of liver lesions. There were umpteen reasons but knowing how luck and fate had dealt blows to me, I was quite confident that it could be a metastasis of my bladder cancer. In layman's terms, my bladder cancer cells would have traveled to the liver and were happily growing there. My friends Sri, Saumya, and Hema came running on hearing the news. If not for friends like this by my side, life would have been tougher.

My doctor advised me to do a PET scan to figure out if the lesion would light up and indeed, it lit up like Christmas lights. We were very confident that the bladder cancer had spread to the liver. My oncologist advised me to talk to a surgeon who can help with removing the tumor. We wanted to get it out fast before thinking of future treatments. Suresh and I downloaded software that can read MRI scans and went through every single picture of the liver where the lesion was seen, researching the cause of liver lesions, and trying to figure out if it was cancer or not. We did not do a biopsy and decided to remove the tumor, as I wanted it out regardless of its malignancy. The fear of cancer forces you to make brave decisions and looming liver surgery does not make one flinch.

The practical part of my brain was thinking about my job. I had just then taken a new job as Director of Test Engineering at a semiconductor firm. *If there was one thing about which I had clarity in my life, it was to ensure that none of my diseases and health struggles define my life.* I never let them stop me from living. At the age of twenty-two, when I was diagnosed with kidney failure, I did not stop going to work and continued until the day of surgery. When diagnosed with cancer at thirty, after the fear had died down, I took a break for three months for chemotherapy and was back the next day.

I changed jobs when I wanted to, to work on what I really like. Going through hurdles in life teaches you what is important. It tells you that if you are delayed getting to work due to a traffic jam, it is ok. It makes you understand that you are lucky for not being the person who met with the accident responsible for the traffic jam. When I was diagnosed with bladder cancer, other than a few weeks leave for surgery, I was at work enjoying what I do. Starting as a junior engineer when diagnosed with kidney failure, to being a director when yet again I was diagnosed with cancer. The standard of my health hurdles seemed to grow with my career.

BE YOUR OWN ADVOCATE

Armed with additional knowledge about the scan, Suresh and I went to the surgeon's office to discuss the surgery. To begin with, the surgeon walked in late and confused me with another patient. Apparently, he had not reviewed the MRI so had no idea where the tumor was in my liver.

When we corrected him, he looked at us condescendingly while telling us not to worry as he knows what he is looking at. Good surgeons generally let you know how they are going to do the surgery, what to look for, how it will feel and when they think you would get better. This surgeon said he must cut through the ribs to reach the liver and remove the tumor even though it was just 1.6 cm. To spice it up, he added that he might actually reach the tumor from the back. When I walked out of the surgeon's office, I had one thought screaming in my head, "Shoba, you have always been your own advocate as an active patient. Is this the surgeon you want?". By evening, I had a clear answer. "No, I will never let my life be dictated by a doctor like that".

GOOD KARMA

After I got home, I called Dr. Sandy at Stanford and asked if she could help me find a surgeon. Over the years, I continued to work with Dr. Sandy by volunteering with the Cancer Institute Foundation (CIF). From my very first cancer diagnosis, I volunteered at CIF helping with their fundraising efforts, most often by organizing various events.

If not for my volunteer work, I may never have had the privilege of having her personal phone number or the courage to call her. In Hinduism, we believe in Karma. As per our scriptures, Karma is the principle of cause and effect that can continue over many lifetimes. I think it was good karma that propelled me to volunteer, thereby getting to know Dr. Sandy.

As soon as she heard about my situation, Dr. Sandy immediately got me an appointment with an excellent surgeon at Stanford, Dr. Visser. I knew I had made the right decision to get a second opinion and if possible, move to a different surgeon. There was a night and day difference when Dr. Visser entered the office. He knew exactly where the tumor was; he drew a picture on a board to show me where the tumor was in my liver. He comforted me saying it was very small and solitary, enabling it to be removed easily. Furthermore, he was very confident that it could be done laparoscopically.

Laparoscopic surgery is a surgical technique in which short, narrow tubes (trocars) are inserted into the abdomen through small (less than one centimeter) incisions. Through these trocars, long, narrow instruments are inserted. The surgeon uses these instruments to manipulate, cut, and sew tissue.

Most patients come out of the surgery with a quick recovery. So far, I had a kidney transplant, TURB, one kidney removal the traditional way with cutting a rib in the process, one kidney removed robotically and a laparoscopic surgery on my liver. What is life if you have not gone through all these surgeries, after all? I always said I was up for a challenge. Never one to be left behind, I realized my body wanted to keep me busy with new challenges.

The surgery was a breeze, and I was able to be back home in three days with just three incisions and a small cut to show I had the surgery. I was lucky and thankful that I decided to go for a second opinion and choose a competent surgeon for the surgery. Imagine my plight if I had gone with the first surgeon who was literally planning to cut me both at the front and the back of my body. If I had not taken the responsibility of what happens to me, I may not have made it out so easily.

For every patient, regardless of the disease, it is very important to get a second opinion. Cancer patients, more so. Most major hospitals and cancer care centers have a separate department for handling second opinions and can be reached easily.

SURPRISING NEWS

When the pathology report came, Dr. Sandy called me to explain. It was a great surprise to learn that the tumor was not a metastasis of my bladder cancer but was a primary tumor of a different cancer called angiosarcoma (AS). Angiosarcoma is a rare cancer that develops in the inner lining of blood vessels and lymph vessels. This cancer can occur anywhere in the body but most often it appears in the skin, breast, liver, and spleen. The news was good and bad. It was good news that I did not have a bladder cancer metastasis, which would have made me a stage 4 patient, statistically with an abysmal prognosis. The bad news was that the cancer was angiosarcoma, an extremely rare aggressive cancer. The good news was my tumor was only 1.6 cm and had not metastasized, so was categorized as a stage 1 cancer.

I was about to let out a sigh when Dr. Sandy said, "Don't google angiosarcoma. It might rattle you. Be strong. We can figure out a plan". I put the phone down and did what a sane person would do in that state. I googled to find out about angiosarcoma of the liver. The sentence that rattled me was: "The prognosis of liver angiosarcoma is very poor with almost all patients with this kind of disease dying within two years after diagnosis". It accounts for 0.1 to 2 percent of all liver malignancies. I had always thought I was a rare breed of human, but this set me miles apart from everyone else.

I cried my heart out while my brain was pondering why I would have gotten this cancer. Could it be the same herb that caused my kidney failure and bladder cancer? Could it be some chemical I have been exposed to? Could it be my lifestyle? Do I need to do something more? I got an appointment with a sarcoma specialist at Stanford, who advised me to undergo an aggressive chemo regimen. She noted that patients who have had extensive chemo tend to fare better for AS.

I consulted with my oncologist Dr. Wu and a sarcoma specialist at Stanford. We finally decided to go for four cycles, with one cycle involving chemo every two weeks, which will essentially take four months to complete. The chemo regimen involved injecting me with docetaxel and gemzar, both drugs with reasonable amount of side effects. I had just then started working at Exar Corporation, a semiconductor firm and this was a setback making me wonder if I had to quit. But my boss was willing to let me work from home. He asked me not to quit but instead continue at my convenience while still managing the team.

SEVERE SIDE EFFECTS

This was not easy at all as it turned out the side effects were quite severe. My body, the one always up for a challenge, was ready once again to go through all the side effects. Severe body pain, nausea, dry eyes resulting in constant tearing, rashes, painful blackened and broken nails, hair loss, low WBC, low RBC, bleeding nose, acidity, burns on my palms, foot, and the skin around the eyes.

The doctors prep you for the therapy with a bunch of drugs readily available for the variety of symptoms:

- Imodium for diarrhea
- Nausea countered by anti-nausea drugs
- MiraLAX for constipation then back to Imodium for diarrhea

- Gargling with salt water for mouth sores
- Neulasta/neupogen shots to increase WBC
- Low RBC/ anemia required a blood transfusion

The one silver lining with this chemo regimen was that it was not toxic to the kidneys. My one transplanted kidney didn't have to take the brunt of a brutal chemo. The other silver lining was that I had gone through chemo before and was a pro at handling side effects. It is a very neat cycle. They give you steroids and anti-nausea drugs before the chemo. The steroids keep you hungry to ensure you are fattening yourself while keeping busy doing all the chores around the house to expend that energy. After a day, the nausea hits you, slowly followed by all the other side effects. By the time the side effects subside, you are ready for the next chemo cycle.

A major difference from my previous chemotherapy was that I had a chemo port installed. A chemo port is a small, implantable reservoir with a thin silicone tube that attaches to a vein. The main advantage of this vein-access device is that chemotherapy medications can be delivered directly into the port rather than a vein, eliminating the need for needle sticks. A life without needle sticks is heaven for a chemo patient albeit a heaven with side effects.

My chemo port was called Betsy, was purple in color, and a cherished friend. I name everything Betsy. My transplanted kidney was also Betsy. I have thousands of surgical clips inside me, and they are all called Betsy.

One might wonder why I was Shoba, and my body parts were Betsy.

Catering to my high standards, my third bout with cancer was a rare and aggressive one with high chances of recurrence. I was not the least bit surprised as it was expected since the standards of my cancers had all been similar. The logical brain could not let it go and wanted

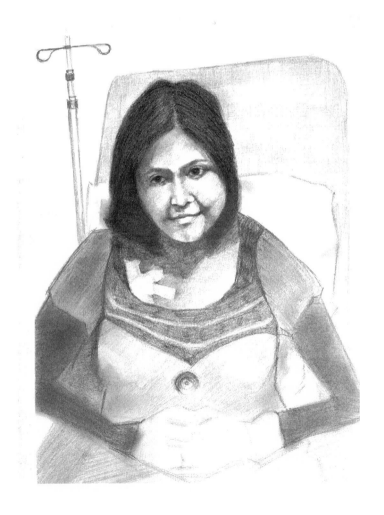

to know why AS found me when it didn't fit my neat theory of kidney failure followed by bladder cancer, due to the ingestion of the herb *aristolochia indica*.

This cancer came out of the blue. "Could it be the herb?" I asked the doctors. "Maybe, maybe not", came their reply. It could also be due to your immunosuppression medications. Compared to facing AS, bladder cancer seemed like child's play. I was alone and couldn't find anyone like me.

FACEBOOK GROUP

I found solace with an AS support group on Facebook. It was started by a couple of AS patients in 2009, with the sole purpose of helping patients find each other because the cancer is so rare and has such a very low remission/cure rate. They had started a non-profit organization to help with research (www.cureasc.org.) Conversing with others in the group gave me a sense of belonging. With renewed energy and optimism, my hopes rose, and I knew I could beat this enemy.

The founder of the group is also a researcher/scientist who is passionately working to find a cure or at least make AS more manageable. The result is a well-connected system of doctors, pathologists, and scientists working on AS, all coming together as a team. In the nine years from my first cancer journey, social media has expanded our world and indeed made the earth feel smaller. The only online group I could find then was a blog called redtoenail.org started by a radiologist as a support group for cancer patients. I was able to make some life-long friends who are alive to date. But, by 2014, our life was filled with Facebook, and everything was at our fingertips. This has helped immensely in the progress of research and support for AS and other cancer patients.

PARTIES

When I found the group, meeting others who were sailing in the same boat as mine, gave me renewed courage and determination. Sharing the chemo experience with others helped me bear the side effects. It was not that bad after all. One week of severe side effects followed by one good week before the next cycle. This gave me courage to plan Suresh's fortieth birthday party. Chemo served as a good camouflage for keeping the party a surprise. Suresh never guessed that I would be throwing a party while undergoing chemo. Being at home, it was easy to organize with the chef and conduct a successful party totally surprising Suresh. Suresh surprised me on my birthday a few months later, along with other friends. Life doesn't wait for anyone to catch up; we must grab it by the hands and keep living despite all the side effects that come along with it.

12 Don't Ask/Please Tell
Be Empathetic

"DO YOU HAVE KIDS?" I was asked.

"When are you planning to have one?" they pressed.

"Don't worry, it all happens in due time," was their sage reply.

I was used to aunties and uncles badgering me with unnecessary, challenging questions on every visit to India. It could even be some random stranger who was sitting next to me on the bus. In India, everyone thinks it is their right to ask prying questions to strangers and our brain is conditioned to that from childhood. But, often, I have seen even the best of the best questioners stumble when it comes to cancer. They give an awkward look trying to convey sympathy with a slight nod conveying, "Oh dear, I understand". Unfortunately, no one understands what a family or a patient goes through while undergoing cancer treatment. Neither the fear of the disease, the pain of the battle, nor the relief of a successful treatment.

"I understand what you are going through." Though this sounds sympathetic, the problem with this comment is that you really don't know what I am going through. Even if you have had cancer yourself, everyone's experience with the disease is different. Some of us breeze through chemo treatments while others suffer a lot, and some don't even make it. I believe that you don't have to try to put yourself in my shoes, as it diminishes what I am going through. The following are suggestions for topics to avoid or pursue with cancer patients, especially me:

Don't ask me questions about my tests. If I want to talk about my blood results, I will. Also, don't ask personal questions that you wouldn't have asked before, especially when it comes to subjects like sex, babies, and religion. Often, though, I have had people getting stumped and blurt out something totally irrelevant to the situation. Coming from India, I am used to people being intrusive, which is one of the reasons why I didn't share my cancer history with friends and family in India for a long time.

Refrain from physical assessments. Refrain from comments about how those with cancer look, particularly if it's negative. And if they just started treatment, don't ask them about potential side effects. If you say anything at all, tell them they look stronger or more beautiful, but mean what you say. I liked it when people complimented me not knowing I was going through chemo or that I was suffering. I could feel it was genuine. But when someone complimented my looks with my blackened eyes and a bald head, it felt insincere maybe, because I was already suffering. "Oh! You are so lucky that your hair grows back so fast. I wish I was as lucky as you", I was told this by one of the receptionists at the hospital. Wow! Lucky me to be able to handle hair loss and go through chemo just because my hair grows back faster.

Don't compare. No, I don't want to know what happened to your friend's friend when she faced cancer. Everyone experiences cancer in his or her own way. Don't bring up the private medical problems of other people you know. I don't want to know about how your friend worked through everything, or how your friend exercised throughout the cancer treatments. Allow me to be who I am. I don't want to be compared to anyone you know. No two cancer patients are alike.

Share encouraging stories. Offer encouragement through success stories of long-term cancer survivors. Avoid saying, "They had the same thing as you." No two cancers are the same. And never tell stories with unhappy endings. If you know someone with the same type of cancer, offer to connect the two of them. Having beaten cancer a few times, my story is encouraging for many patients. I have always been happy to share and help them overcome their battle having sailed the same sea. The worst example would be talking about someone who succumbed to the disease, I still remember one of my colleagues talking about his grandfather's skin cancer, the day I went back to work after one of my surgeries. He went into great length about how his grandfather went through surgery but finally died after none of the treatments helped. That was not really the encouragement I was looking for.

Show them you care. Show those with cancer that they're loved. Give them a hug. Surprise them with books, magazines, or music. Asking an open-ended question like "How can I help you?" is not going to really help. A cancer patient would neither have the energy nor the mental clarity to ask you to run an errand—everyone has their own priorities. Be specific by asking, "What day can I bring you dinner?" And offer to help only if you intend to follow through with it and won't expect something in return. When I was undergoing chemo, my friend Devi offered to bring me fresh home-cooked lunch to my workplace, for one week. It was not even a question. She decided to help and informed me that she will be providing my lunch. That is the kind of friend one would want to be. We have had friends who were ready to stay at the hospital so Suresh could take a break. They all helped purely out of love and concern.

Don't trivialize their experience. Try not to say, "Don't worry, you'll be fine." You don't know that. These statements downplay what she is going through. Instead say, "I'm really sorry," or "I hope it will be okay." I hated it from the bottom of my heart and still do today, when someone says, "Don't worry, everything will be fine." I felt as though they were jinxing my life. It is so irritating to hear people say that especially when they don't have any idea of what I am going through. When I got cancer at thirty, some nurses responded with, "It is good to get cancer at a young age as your body can handle the treatments better". I sincerely cannot make up my mind as to whether they were apathetic or trying to help.

There is no good cancer. Don't refer to the patient's cancer as "the good cancer." There is no such thing as a good cancer. Is there really a "good" kind of cancer? Leave the door to communication open so they can talk about fears and concerns.

It is not about you. Avoid talking about your headache, backache, etc. This isn't about you. And as bad as you feel, he or she feels worse and may not be interested in hearing about how hard this has been on your life. Don't put him or her in the position of having to comfort you. Only ask questions if you truly want to hear the response. There have been many instances where I have had to comfort my friends on mundane issues while going through side effects of chemo.

Think before you speak. Your words and actions can be powerful. Avoid clichés, like "hero" and "battle." If the person gets worse, does it mean they didn't fight hard enough? Don't make it sound as though the cancer was fully under the person's control and somehow, they screwed it up. "Maybe you should have exercised more/eaten more vegetables, etc." Comments like these and "How did you get it?" sound suspiciously like blame and imply that the person who got cancer is at fault. The last thing you want to do is blame someone who is dealing with such a difficult experience.

When one of my friends heard I got cancer for the second time, her response was one of anger. "I have told you not to get stressed about things. Look what happened.

You should have never left meditating". The barrage of thoughts continued while I was crying on the other end. She did apologize later. It was her way of processing but unfortunately one that doesn't help. While undergoing treatment, a friend said, "At least you know when you are going to die so you can plan accordingly". As much as that might sound practical, death is terrifying, and no one wants to face it unless they are terminal and in hospice. You must be sensitive. As much as the intellectual brain understands death might be forthcoming, the heart never loses hope.

Don't ignore. Some people disappear when someone they know gets cancer. The worst thing you can do is avoid the person because you don't know how to handle it. Cancer is a lonely disease and isolating as it is. Tell them, "I'm here for you." Just stay connected. Luckily for me, every single close friend of mine has stayed connected and, along with my family, has never left my side. The ones who lost touch never mattered anyway.

13 One More Lap of the Race
Make A Plan

"I AM SORRY, SHOBA. It seems to have returned."

We were at the doctor's office for a follow-up. After my remission from angiosarcoma, there was a small but ever-present, lesion in my liver which showed up in every follow up albeit with a very, very slow growth. It was thought to be something benign and not to worry about, but my oncologist was monitoring it in every follow-up. On one of my appointments, she asked me to check with my surgeon. Since I was on a three-month follow-up schedule then, the scans were quite frequent and in December of 2015 when the growth went past one centimeter Dr. Visser, my surgeon gave me the bad news that it might be time to take out the lesion.

I was not ready. Suresh was not ready. My body was not ready. My brain and heart were not ready for the news. And the tears came streaming down my cheeks again. We drove back home and informed our friends. It was *deja vu* all over again, for me, for Suresh, for my family and for my friends.

It was just one year from the end of my chemo treatments. I went into a state of panic not knowing how to deal with this blow. AS is known to be very aggressive with a high recurrence rate but the little voice within me always gave me hope that I could be in that one percent who survive AS. Maybe, it was not destined to be. The fact that there was a recurrence within one year would mean the chemo treatment did not work. That was the thought that made me panic even more as I was used to fighting the disease because there was hope at the end of it all.

Dr. Visser spoke to the sarcoma specialist at Stanford, Dr. Ganjoo who had consulted with my oncologist for my treatment of AS a year before. She gave us hope that after surgery, we could try some novel treatments that have become available. The plan was to have surgery, followed by some treatments. I was afraid to do a biopsy because if it were AS, it is a cancer that occurs in blood vessels, and there could be every chance it spreads once pierced with a needle. Since this lesion was present for more than a year, the assumption was that it would be AS that was missed before and one that chemo did not fight.

BE YOUR OWN ADVOCATE

My immediate thought was to get a second opinion from a well-known doctor who has worked solely on AS and has treated many AS patients. I sent all my documents to his clinic and waited eagerly for his opinion. The speed with which he called me impressed me a lot. I got a call at 8:00 a.m. in the morning from the specialist. He advised me to go through chemo therapies first to shrink and kill the tumor, followed by surgery to remove it.

He was very concerned especially since it was AS of the liver for which the survival rate is almost nil. The protocol to administer chemotherapy first followed by surgery is followed only by a few oncologists, whereas surgical removal was the gold standard. I listened to him patiently and told him that I will consider the option. This got me terribly confused as to which way to proceed. If we had done a biopsy, it would have told us if the tumor was indeed AS but since this cancer occurs in the blood vessels, a biopsy with a needle might actually spread it faster.

After much consultation with Dr. Sandy, who has been my guide, we decided to go ahead with the surgery. There was still a lot of confusion in my mind until the very last minute. On the day I was ready to let the surgeon know about my decision, I got in touch with Corrie Painter, a scientist and an AS survivor from our Facebook group and brainstormed with her about my predicament. She immediately put me in touch with another AS specialist who advised me to follow what Dr. Ganjoo had suggested which was surgery. I received opinions from three doctors, consulted with one more, and finally came to the decision to continue with surgery first, right before entering the exam room to consult with my surgeon.

MONDAY SURGERY

If all my previous surgeries had taught me something, it was the foresight to schedule the surgery on a Monday so that I will have the surgeon and other doctors available through the week instead of struggling to find them over the weekend. This was an open liver surgery from which I was wheeled out somewhere around midnight after getting into the surgical room in the morning. The whole right lobe of my liver had to come out as the lesion was embedded deep in a hard-to-reach location. When I was wheeled into my room, Suresh bent down and whispered, "The doctor took it all out and says he could not find the exact location of the tumor. It looks different than before". Suresh knew I would be eager to know about the outcome even if I was half conscious. And I surely did appreciate knowing before promptly falling asleep.

With a bruised abdomen, I was barely able to get up from the bed when on day three after the surgery, I was feeling very dizzy and knew deep inside that something was terribly wrong. I had not passed urine for the past two days and I could see that my bag was empty. As it happens in university hospitals, I was constantly visited by multitude of fellows and residents to whom Suresh had to answer the same set of questions every single time, much to his chagrin.

NEW ISSUE

That morning, the ICU nurses were waiting to shift me to ICU as I was close to a code blue. Apparently, my liver was still healing hence not working well and my transplanted kidney had shut down. My hemoglobin levels were very low indicating I might need blood. But my surgeon hesitated to give me blood as I was a kidney recipient, and he was not sure how the immune system would react to the transfusion.

That evening, I was barely able to stay awake when one of the senior nephrologists visited me. He was informed of my situation by my nephrologist to ensure the treatments at the hospital does not interfere with my transplant. When he came in, he had one look at my blood pressure which was very low and got concerned. "Please help me, Doc", I pleaded. He immediately called my surgeon who was performing a surgery and advised him to administer a blood transfusion.

Throughout the day, with people walking in and out of the room, Suresh was getting frustrated, panicked, and stressed that no action was being taken. Finally, by evening, one bottle of blood was given which helped my blood pressure and I opened my eyes to see our friends also standing by my bed along with Suresh.

The nurses were about to administer the second bag when I noticed that it was B-. The first question that I asked when I woke up was to the nurse, "I am B+. Why are you administering B- blood?" Suresh, Sri, and Hema, who were in the room were astonished that they didn't notice it. As I always say, "Be your own advocate." This is a story that is regaled by all of us on how alert I was even when I was close to losing my life. As a side note, patients with B+ blood can be given B- blood. I clearly insisted the nurses give me B+ blood which was my right as a patient; I demanded B+ blood and they changed the bags.

EARLY CHRISTMAS GIFT

That night, the day before Christmas Eve, was the most crucial night in my recovery. A nurse was assigned specifically to look after me. She was present in my room throughout the night monitoring my kidney function. Suresh slept fitfully nearby. Slowly, my one transplanted kidney, fondly called Betsy, came back to life much to everyone's delight. This was my own sweet little Christmas gift to myself. This was a surgery which made me feel as though I was teasing death into coming back to life. I attained Nirvana that night.

I was discharged a couple of days later and had a slow recovery for the next couple of weeks while my liver was healing. While reading the discharge papers, I found that I got a buy one, get one offer without my knowledge. Along with the right lobe of my liver, my gallbladder was also removed. None of us had a clue until reading the discharge papers that day. It was done and dusted so nothing more could be done—my gallbladder was gone.

WHAT A RELIEF

The ancient Greek myth of Titan Prometheus and his punishment for deceiving Zeus and protecting mankind is known to most members of the scientific community who study hepatic diseases, mainly because Prometheus' liver was the target of torture. However, the myth of Prometheus is known and cherished by many, because, according to one version, Prometheus created the first man. The ancient poet Hesiod (8th century BC) records that Prometheus twice tricked the gods.

First, he offered mortals the best meat from a slaughtered cow and gave the fat and bones to the gods. Then, when an infuriated Zeus punished man by taking fire, Prometheus stole it back for mankind. Accordingly, Zeus punished him in two ways. First, Prometheus was bound on the mountain Caucasus. More explicitly, for students of the liver, an eagle fed from his liver each day, but the liver regenerated overnight. Well, it is not just Prometheus's liver that regenerated overnight, human livers do too albeit a bit more slowly. The only organ in our body that can grow back to full function after being cut, is the liver.

With the torture my liver had gone through, I was eagerly waiting for the pathology report to know what I was dealing with, but it was taking unusually long. Unable to curtail myself, I texted Dr. Sandy and asked her if she had any information. A slight hope blossomed when she said that the first pathology report from the pathologist claimed that the cells were not malignant.

I was getting restless that the official report was taking forever and started calling the surgeon's office every day. Finally, one of the nurses called me back and explained that two pathologists had different views and the tumor sample was sent to Harvard to get a third opinion from a renowned pathologist there. On my follow-up visit, it was proclaimed that the cells were atypical but not malignant. I was not sure how to react. Should I be relieved that it was not cancer, or should I feel foolish that I went ahead with a complicated surgery which pulled me close to death? I had mixed feelings, ones of relief, elation, and guilt in case I had died. Relief of not having cancer, elation that I didn't have to go through brutal treatments, and guilt that I might have left Suresh alone if I had died in the process.

REMISSION

My race for life has been going on from that day through now. I am running, evading, and always trying to be one step ahead so that the beast can never catch me—I am counting on many more years of life. To give myself the best chance for survival, nutrition is important to me. I am sharing a few of my favorite dishes and recipes in the next chapter.

14 Nutrition

FROM MY FIRST STINT with cancer, I have been very conscious of what goes into my body. Being an Indian has made consuming some of the superfoods quite easy as most of them play a traditional role in Indian cuisine.

MAITAKE MUSHROOM:

Maitake (grifola frondose) is a type of mushroom. It forms large clumps on tree stumps and tree roots. It was first used in traditional Asian medicine.

The maitake mushroom grows in forests in Asia, Europe, and eastern North America. It contains chemicals that might help fight tumors, stimulate the immune system, and lower blood sugar levels. A key component in maitake mushrooms is beta-glucan, a type of polysaccharide, a long molecule of carbohydrates found to affect the immune system.

Beta glucan is a soluble fiber that provides digestive benefits and may boost immune function. Maitake is even being researched as a potential cancer-fighter. In laboratory research, scientists have found that maitake extracts may slow the growth of certain tumors. By spurring activity in immune cells (such as natural killer cells and T-cells), maitake is thought to help inhibit the growth of cancer cells. A component of beta-glucan known as the D-fraction has been found to have anti-tumor activity.[7]

I did not grow up eating mushrooms and hence acquiring that taste took a while, but this curry recipe infuses the flavor of ginger with the mushrooms and enhances the taste.

MAITAKE MUSHROOM CURRY

Ingredients
¼ cup shredded fresh coconut
1 inch of a green chili (serrano or jalapeno)
cumin seeds
2-inch-long piece of ginger
1 tsp. turmeric powder
1 pound maitake mushrooms
1 tbsp. olive oil
1 tsp. salt (as needed)

Cooking Method
1. Clean the mushrooms by rubbing the dirt off with a brush or rinsing them quickly under running water. Do not soak them in water for long as they tend to become soggy. Cut into uniformly thin slices.

2. Crush or blend coarsely ginger, coconut, cumin, and chili

3. In a pan, pour the oil and sauté the above blended paste with turmeric powder. After a minute, add the mushrooms. Mushrooms have a ton of water in them, which seeps out while cooking. Keep the flame on medium high heat. Don't cover the pan. Stir it every two minutes. Add salt.

4. Make sure that the water has evaporated. Taste the mushrooms and add more salt if desired. Add chopped cilantro as garnish.

CARROTS:

One of the easiest vegetables to love, carrots are packed with disease-fighting nutrients. They contain beta-carotene, an antioxidant scientists believe may protect cell membranes from toxin damage and slow the growth of cancer cells. And carrots deliver other vitamins and phytochemicals that might guard against cancers of the mouth, esophagus, and stomach. Some studies suggest carrots protect against cervical cancer, perhaps because they supply antioxidants that could battle HPV (human papilloma virus), the major cause of cervical cancer. Plus, carrots contain falcarinol, a natural pesticide.[8]

CARROT, MOONG SPROUTS SALAD

Ingredients
    1 pound carrots
    1 cup moong sprouts
    1 inch of a green chili
    1 inch piece of ginger
    1 tsp. cumin
    1 tsp. mustard
    1 tbsp. olive oil
    1 tsp. lemon juice

Cooking Method

1. Dice green chili and ginger.

2. In a pan, sauté the mustard, cumin, diced chili, and ginger until the mustard seeds splutter.

3. Grate the carrots and mix with moong sprouts, mix in the above sauteed items with the oil. Add salt and lemon juice. Mix and serve.

BROCCOLI:

Broccoli sprouts are young broccoli plants that have high amounts of glucoraphanin, a precursor of sulforaphane. Sulforaphane is a sulfur-rich compound known to benefit human health.

Sulforaphane may block the initiation stage in carcinogenesis by inhibiting enzymes that convert procarcinogens to carcinogens and inducing phase two enzymes that metabolize carcinogens to facilitate excretion. Induction of phase 2 enzymes occurs through antioxidant response element-driven gene expression, with targets including NAD(P)H: quinone reductase, heme oxygenase 1, and gamma-glutamylcysteine synthetase regulated by nuclear factor E2 related factor. Sulforaphane also suppresses cancer development through various molecular targets. It induces G2/M cell cycle arrest via cyclin-dependent kinases and triggers dose-dependent apoptosis and inhibits histone deacetylase by its metabolites in vitro.

Broccoli sprouts have also been investigated for their potential anticancer properties. Preclinical studies suggest sulforaphane may have anticancer effects against prostate, breast and urinary cancers and may also protect skin from ultraviolet radiation.[9]

When I was diagnosed with bladder cancer, broccoli was the go-to food almost every other day as it is proven to help urinary cancers. This simple sprout sandwich is quite filling.

BROCCOLI SPROUTS SANDWICH

Ingredients

½ cup broccoli sprouts
6 avocado slices
1 tsp. cumin powder
1 tsp. black pepper powder
1 tsp. lemon juice
Salt as per preference
2 slices of whole wheat bread or Ezekiel sprouted bread
¼ cup shredded cheese (vegan cheese if you are vegan)

Cooking Method

1. Toast the bread slices.

2. Layer in the following order:

3. Toast—shredded cheese—avocado slices—broccoli sprouts—salt with cumin and pepper powder—lemon juice—avocado slices—cheese—toast

LENTILS:

Lentils are a nutrient powerhouse, loaded with protein, fiber, and a whole range of micronutrients, one of them being iron. Just a half-cup serving of lentils packs almost 20 percent of your daily iron needs. If you're not used to eating lentils or don't know where to start, they are a great addition to soups and stews, curries, and even burgers.[10]

When I was going through chemotherapy, my iron levels started dipping quite low and the nurse recommended an iron supplement. For a vegetarian, lentils are a boon as they cover a whole range of nutrients usually found in meat. These lentil balls are the best bet to get some protein while recuperating.

STEAMED LENTIL BALLS

½ cup toor dal (Indian Lentil)
½ cup chana dal (Indian Lentil)
water (for soaking)
½ cup coconut (grated)
3 tbsp. dill leaves (finely chopped)
2 tbsp. cilantro (finely chopped)
A few curry leaves (chopped—optional, if available)
1 inch piece of ginger (finely chopped)
1 tsp. cayenne pepper powder
1 tsp. cumin / jeera
A pinch of asafetida
¾ tsp. salt

Cooking Method

1. In a bowl place ½ cup toor dal and ½ cup chana dal. Add enough water and soak for three hours.

2. Drain the lentils and transfer to a food processor. Blend to a coarse paste without adding any water.

3. Put the coarse paste of lentils into a large bowl.

4. Add ½ cup coconut, 3 tbsp. dill leaves, 2 tbsp. coriander and a few curry leaves.

5. Also add ginger, chili, cumin and ¾ tsp. salt. Squeeze and mix well until all the spices are combined well.

6. Grease your hand with oil and form a cylindrical shape.

7. Place in a steamer leaving enough space in between. Steam for 15 to 20 minutes or until the balls are cooked completely.

The Indian lentils can be substituted with split lentils of any kind that is available.

WHOLE GRAINS:

Whole grains are a great source of fiber. Dietary fiber can help you maintain a healthy weight and help lower your cancer risk. People often assume the only whole grain available is whole wheat. I always read the nutrition/ingredients label when looking for foods containing whole grains. Any food with the following will be categorized as a whole grain: brown rice, buckwheat, bulgur, millet, oatmeal, rolled oats, whole grain barley, whole grain corn, whole grain sorghum, whole oats, whole rye, wild rice. I personally favor millets, quinoa, oats, and brown rice. Here is a millet porridge recipe which is comforting especially during therapy.

MILLET PORRIDGE

Ingredients

½ cup Foxtail millets

½ cup quinoa

½ cup split lentils (any kind)

5 cups water

1 cup diced veggies (carrots, string beans, bell peppers, cabbage, broccoli, peas)

1.5 tbsp. ghee (clarified butter—can be replaced with oil)

1 tsp. grated ginger

½ tsp. cumin

¼ tsp. cayenne pepper

½ tsp. turmeric

salt as needed

Cooking Method

1. Wash millet, quinoa, and lentils in water. Soak for an hour. Drain.

2. In a pot, add the ghee. When the ghee is hot, set heat to low and add a teaspoon of cumin seeds.

3. As soon as the cumin seeds crackle put the washed millets, quinoa, and lentils along with the veggies into the pan.

4. Stir for a minute, then add turmeric, cayenne pepper, salt and five cups of water.

5. Bring to a boil.

6. Set heat to low, cover the pan and let it simmer. Check the pan after fifteen minutes to stir and add more water if you want the dish soupier.

7. Continue to cook for about twenty-five minutes, or till the millets and lentils have softened and come together. Let the pan stand covered for another ten minutes.

8. The porridge is ready.

GARLIC:

Garlic has benefits that go beyond flavoring food. It contains antibacterial and antioxidant properties. It has also been linked to a reduced risk of developing certain cancers. Garlic has natural antioxidants and is an anti-inflammatory, antibacterial, and antiviral food. It contains high levels of sulfur, flavonoids, and selenium. And, when it is crushed, chopped, or bruised, garlic produces the compound allicin.[11] I tend to crush or chop garlic and leave it in the open for ten minutes before cooking them.

Garlic has some key cancer fighting compounds:

- Allicin: This is a powerful plant compound that is antibiotic (substance that inhibits or kills microorganisms) and antifungal (inhibits growth of fungi). Raw is best since cooking speeds the breakdown of allicin, and microwaving appears to kill it and destroy the health benefits.

- Flavonoids: These are aromatic plant compounds that are considered to have antioxidant (prevents or slows the damage to cells caused by free radicals) and anti-inflammatory (prevents or reduces inflammation) properties. These compounds fight cancer by preventing cell damage.

- Selenium and allyl sulfides: These substances keep cell DNA from being damaged, which can prevent the development of cancer.[12]

Onions, garlic, and ginger are a staple in Indian cuisine. In our household, while growing up, my mom never cooked with garlic as she was not fond of the flavor. In my 30s, after my first bout of cancer, I started eating garlic and it has become a staple today.

GARLIC PEPPER SOUP

This soup is tangy, spicy, and heavenly. It is loaded with the goodness of tomatoes, pepper, and garlic.

Ingredients

10 grams tamarind soaked in 1 cup water and squeezed to get tamarind juice

5 to 6 cloves garlic peeled and 1 crushed

1 to 2 chopped tomatoes (medium size)

Salt as required

For grinding into a powder:

1 tsp. whole black pepper

1 tsp. cumin seeds

1 clove garlic (optional)

For the seasoning:

1 tsp. ghee

½ tsp. black mustard seeds

½ tsp. cumin/jeera seeds

A few curry leaves

For garnishing:

Coriander leaves – finely chopped

Cooking Method

1. Take the squeezed 1 cup tamarind extract and add chopped tomatoes, salt, curry leaves, whole peeled garlic, 1 clove crushed garlic and the coarsely ground powder of pepper and cumin.

2. Boil over low flame until it reduces a little and the raw smell of the tamarind goes away.

3. Then add 1 1/2-1 3/4 cups of water. When you see froth forming on the surface, switch off the stove. The soup is ready.

4. Heat a tsp of ghee, add mustard seeds, cumin seeds, then when it crackles, add curry leaves, and pour it over the soup.

5. Garnish with finely chopped coriander leaves.

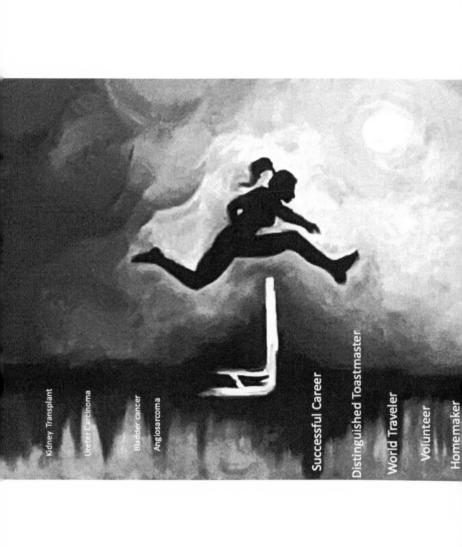

Kidney Transplant

Ureter Carcinoma

Bladder cancer

Angiosarcoma

Successful Career

Distinguished Toastmaster

World Traveler

Volunteer

Homemaker

15 The Fight Continues
I Am Not My Disease

ALL OUR MOTOR skills are stored in our brain. We never think about how our body moves, eats, or performs various functions. When cancer strikes, the same body that you trusted has produced cells that are ready to kill you. The horrors of chemo, surgery, hospitalization, and everything that is thrown at you with the aim of making you better, breaks you physically and mentally. You finally beat the disease and are given a "no evidence of disease" stamp. You are clearly told that the word "cure" is a taboo and is never uttered. The closest you can get to being cured is not showing evidence of disease in your body. The same body that you trusted would be fine because you ate healthy and always strived hard to keep fit.

It would be so amazing if you were cured, and you couldn't get it again. Some people go through their entire lives without knowing the meaning of cancer and worrying only about simple chronic conditions. You wish and ache to be that person. The odds of being struck by cancer again seem higher. The fear never goes away. Every "No evidence of disease" brings you momentary happiness. It is a race for your life.

I AM NOT MY DISEASE

Should this bring down your morale? Should that stop you from living? Many patients suffer from post-traumatic stress disorder (PTSD) but it is up to all of us to overcome the stress and not let the disease define who we are. As I often say, "I am not the disease". I don't want to be known as Shoba, the cancer survivor. I am a daughter, a wife, a successful career woman, a world traveler, a toastmaster, a volunteer, a friend, a sister, godmother to two children, a daughter-in-law and above all a confident, brave woman. No cancer can change that. The most important lesson I have learned over the decade is not to let any disease define my life but to *live life* to the fullest extent, with the disease as a blip in a corner, albeit traveling with me.

Every time cancer struck, we faced it bravely and gave a good fight. But that did not stop us from living. I graduated with a Masters in electrical engineering from Stanford University one year after my first cancer bout. My husband Suresh and I have traveled to at least fifteen countries and various states in the US. We have enjoyed every moment in our lives and created a lot of cherished memories one day at a time. As the phrase goes, "Life is a dance, so let your feet up". We danced merrily to life's tunes and had the time of our life during our travels. We have visited countries all the way from Asia to the Americas. Trying to find the right bus to go back to our hotel in Rome to time spent with a Japanese geisha, we have built lots of memories. Visiting countries like Iceland

and New Zealand, lands of raw nature, has filled us with eternal calm and made us realize that this life exists for a reason, and we should not skimp on it or forget to live due to a disease. Never let the disease consume you.

At every juncture when faced with the mountain of hardship, I have often wondered if I should quit working. But then I wonder what I would do. I cannot think of me being anything other than a career woman. I have had major health struggles, starting from my kidney failure within two years into my career, continuing with various hiccups every five to six years. I have had a successful career span of twenty-six years with no major break due to pure grit and determination.

Support from coworkers, friends and family kept me going though it was very tough attending work with all the side effects of chemo. It is indeed uncomfortable to listen to mandatory harassment training while your whole body is screaming in pain. Starting my career as an analog engineer in a semiconductor world filled with only men, I am thankful and proud that I have been able to weave through all the hurdles and be a successful leader today. Being financially independent, I have been able to support my parents while traveling around the world taking them to visit a variety of places.

GIVING BACK

Many cancer patients find peace in helping with research and giving back to the cancer community. I am no different. As soon as I finished my chemotherapy in 2005, I badly wanted to help cancer patients in some way. That is when I met Kannan, who had started a 501C3 nonprofit organization in California, to raise funds for the Cancer Institute (WIA), a cancer hospital that was giving free cancer care for poor patients in the region. https://cancerinstitutewia.in/CI-WIA/

It has been serving the community since 1954 when it was started by Dr. Muthulakshmi Reddy, a true feminist and the first woman doctor of India. From December 2005 to today, I have been volunteering for this organization in raising funds at various events, using my public speaking skills, acting as the master of ceremonies for all our events. When I was diagnosed with angiosarcoma, I found support with Angiosarcoma Awareness (https://www.cureasc.org/) and have been trying my best to help them with their research.

Every day is filled with gratitude for all these institutions that have been formed with the sole intention of helping others. It was a proud and slightly embarrassing moment when one of my friends nominated me to receive an award from our local congressman for community service. If there is one thing I don't know how to handle is praise in any form, especially for helping others.

Often, many cancer patients become depressed, suffering from PTSD. I have been able to find a window to the outside world via Toastmasters. Toastmasters is an organization formed to help people with public speaking and leadership skills. Being a member for eleven years now, I have delivered lots of speeches, thereby venting my heart out, meeting new people, hearing different perspectives, mentoring many to become good leaders and speakers. When you hear a different perspective, your situation feels small and bearable. There is inspiration in each speech I have heard and every person I have met.

Don't put me in a box. My mantra is: "I am not my disease." I am a wife, a daughter, a friend, an engineer, and a woman of my own making.

My body feels weak, my spirit's not strong
My race against death, feels so long
My fears and doubts, they come and go
But I must keep running, if I'm to grow

I am not my disease, it will not define me
My strength and resilience, you will soon see
I am not my disease,I will not be a slave
My mind and soul, I will bravely save.

My faith and courage, they shall not wane
My race against death, I must sustain
Though I'm tired and weary, I keep pushing on
My race against death, I'm determined to win

Acknowledgments

Writing a book is lot harder and takes longer than I thought. It is lot more rewarding once done with a renewed sense of purpose. None of this would have been possible without the encouragement of my family and friends. I must start by thanking my awesome husband, Suresh, who has helped me from reading the very early drafts to advising me at every step of the book's writing, editing, and publishing, while also sketching the illustrations.. Thank you so much, dear.

To my mother, Ramamani, who has given me a second chance at life and has been with me throughout my journey. Thank you from the bottom of my heart. To my father, Keshava Rao, who has been my role model; thank you for inculcating valuable principles and virtues in me.

To my two sisters, Uma and Hema, who helped me relive my childhood and ensured the details are accurate. Thank you for being the ever-supportive sisters.

I am eternally grateful to all my doctors who have helped me survive to write this book. If not for the timely decisions and advice from you all, I may not be living to see this day. A special thanks to Dr. Sandy, who guided me during some of my toughest times.

Thanks to my numerous colleagues who have been there when needed, covering for me, and letting me take breaks to deal with my health struggles.

A very special thanks to my friends Sri, Hema, and

Karthi, who have encouraged me in all my ventures. To my friends Saumya and Susheela, who took the time to review the manuscript and recommend suggestions to make the content flow better—thank you.

Lastly, the book would not be possible if not for Henry DeVries and team at Indie Books International who guided me through the editing and publishing process. Thanks to Lisa Lucas, who meticulously helped me edit and convert the book into meaningful chapters. To Devin DeVries, thank you for helping with the publishing.

About The Author

Shoba Rao was born and raised in a middle-class family along with her two sisters, in the southern part of India. She moved to the Bay Area in 2000 after her marriage to her husband, Suresh, who was brave enough to marry her despite the idiosyncrasies. They currently live amidst the mountains and valleys of Bay Area, California. She is an engineer at heart and has a masters in electrical engineering from Stanford University. She is a successful career woman with twenty-five years of experience in the semiconductor industry and currently serves as director of manufacturing engineering. In her spare time, she enjoys exercising, reading books, dancing, painting, baking, cooking, and volunteering with various organizations.

Shoba is a three-time cancer survivor and a kidney transplant recipient. The idea of this book originated when many friends came to her seeking for advice when a loved one or a friend got afflicted with cancer or any other major disease. Her passion to serve the community inspired her to write this book with the hope of helping others.

She is a Distinguished Toastmaster and often shares her life journey in various speeches, focusing on inspirational speeches with a humorous touch. She is passionate about mentoring others and conducts workshops on many subjects. She is open to speaking opportunities about her book with the hope that it can serve as an inspiration and motivate the audience to live life to the fullest.

Endnotes

1   *Digsby, the Biggest Dog in the World,* directed by Joseph McGrath, written by Charles Isaacs, Ted Key, and Michael Pertwee, (London, UK: City Investing Company--Walter Shenson Films, 1974)

2   *Goldeneye,* directed by Martin Campbell, written by Ian Fleming, Michael France , Jeffrey Caine, and Bruce Feinstein (London, UK: Eon Productions, United Artists, 1995).

3   Eliyahi M. Goldratt and Jeff Cox, *The Goal: The Process of Ongoing Improvement,* (Great Barrington, MA: North River Press, 2014)

4   Frédéric D.Debelle Jean-Louis Vanherweghem,¹and Joëlle L.Nortier, "Aristolochic Acid Nephrology: A Worldwide Problem", *ScienceDirect,* July 2, 2008, Accessed June 7, 2022, https://www.sciencedirect.com/science/article/pii/S0085253815532791)

5   Jimi Yoon, Young-Woo Sun, and Tae-Heung Kim, "Complementary and Alternative Medicine for Vitiligo", White-Line Skin Clinic & Research Center, Kyungnam Republic of Korea, 2011, Chapter 3.2 Accessed June 7, 2022, https://cdn.intechopen.com/pdfs/24976/intech-complementary_and_alternative_medicine_for_vitiligo.pdf.

6   Nikola M. Pavlovic, "Balkan endemic nephropathy—current status and future perspectives", *National Library of Medicine,* June 3, 2013, Accessed June 7, 2022, https://www.ncbi.nlm.nih.gov/pmc/articles/PMC4400492/

7   T. Soussi, "The p53 tumor suppressor gene: from molecular biology to clinical investigation", *National Library of Medicine,* June 9, 2000, Accessed June 7, 2022. https://pubmed.ncbi.nlm.nih.gov/10911910/

8   Frank Herbert, *Dune,* (Boston, MA: Chilton Books, 1965)

9   Noriko Kodama, Kiyoshi Komuta, and Hiroaki Nanba, "Effect of Maitake (Grifola frondosa) D-Fraction on the activation of NK cells in cancer patients", *National Library of Medicine*, Winter 2003, Accessed June 7, 2022, "https://pubmed.ncbi.nlm.nih.gov/14977447/

10 "Falcarinol, a Compound in Carrots- Could Reduce Cancer Risk", Carrotmuseum.com, Accessed June 7, 2022, http://www.carrotmuseum.co.uk/falcarinol.html

11 D.B. Nandini, Roopa S. Rao, B.S. Deepak, and Praveen B. Reddy, "Sulforaphane in broccoli: The green chemoprevention!! Role in cancer prevention and therapy", *National Library of Medicine*, May-August 2020, Accessed June 7, 2022, https://www.ncbi.nlm.nih.gov/pmc/articles/PMC7802872/

12 Lentils.org https://www.lentils.org/health-nutrition/nutritional-information/

13 Leyla Bayan, Peir Hossain Koulivand, and Ali Gorji, "Garlic, a review of potential therapeutic effects", National Library of Medicine, January-February 2014, Accessed June 7, 2022, https://www.ncbi.nlm.nih.gov/pmc/articles/PMC4103721/ J.A. Milner, "A Historical Perspective on Garlic and Cancer," *The Journal of Nutrition*, March 2001, Accessed June 7, 2022, https://academic.oup.com/jn/article/131/3/1027S/4687047

13 *Goldeneye*, directed by Martin Campbell, written by Ian Fleming, Michael France , Jeffrey Caine, and Bruce Feinstein (London, UK: Eon Productions, United Artists, 1995).

NOTES

NOTES

NOTES